Are You In A Co-dependent Relationship?

- Do you feel rejected when your partner is spending time with friends?
- Do you feel shame when your partner makes a mistake?
- Do you have sex when you don't want to?
- Do you keep silent in order to keep the peace?
- Do you feel like you give and give and get little or no return?

These are just some of the questions in the Co-dependency Relationship Questionnaire on page 7 which will help you determine whether or not your sexual relationships are, or have been, co-dependent. *Healing Together* tells you why you keep finding yourself in dysfunctional and painful relationships, and gives a concrete course of action for moving toward healthy sexual relationships.

Wayne Kritsberg gives lectures and workshops throughout the country in the areas of intimacy, healing childhood sexual abuse, co-dependency, adult children of alcoholics issues and spirituality. For information about his workshops and audiotapes call (512) 327-4130 in Austin, Texas.

HEALING TOGETHER

A Guide To Intimacy And Recovery For Co-dependent Couples

Wayne Kritsberg

Health Communications, Inc.
Deerfield Beach, Florida

Wayne Kritsberg
Austin, Texas

Library of Congress Cataloging-in-Publication Data

Kritsberg, Wayne
    Healing together: a guide to intimacy and recovery for co-dependent
    couples/Wayne Kritsberg.
       p.   cm.
    Includes bibliographical references.
    ISBN 1-55874-053-8: $8.95
    1. Co-dependence (Psychology)   2. Interpersonal relations.
    3. Intimacy (Psychology) I. Title.
RC569.5.C63K75   1989   89-39226
158'.24—dc20   CIP

©1990 Wayne Kritsberg
ISBN 1-55874-053-8

Publisher: Health Communications, Inc.
               3201 S.W. 15th Street
               Deerfield Beach, Florida 33442

Dedicated to
Ceci, my life partner, and
Matthew, my son and newest teacher.

Acknowledgments

I would like to thank the former clients who confided in me and who provided the personal information and stories contained in this book. Without their inspirational courage to recover from co-dependence, this book would not have been possible.

A special thanks and appreciation must go to my wife Ceci Miller-Kritsberg, a poet and writer, who edited this book. She took the raw manuscript and turned it into a readable book. Ceci's contributions to this work, however, were more than the long hours she spent editing; she also contributed important original ideas and insights that became an integral part of this work. Her loving support and gentle editorial guidance helped to turn the difficult task of writing into a healing experience. Ceci is a truly remarkable woman, and I am blessed to have her as my life partner. Thank you, Ceci, for your help, guidance and understanding. Without you this book would be much less than it is.

I would also like to thank my Higher Power for the gift of recovery, and for the unconditional love and guidance I have received throughout my life.

The examples used in this book are based upon actual case histories of co-dependents who are in the process of recovery. In order to insure privacy and confidentiality, I have either changed the names of the persons in the example or have created composites of different case histories.

Contents

Introduction

Living in a co-dependent relationship means living in pain and frustration. As a counselor and lecturer, I have met and worked with many co-dependents who struggle in their sexual relationships. Many of them have wandered from one disastrous relationship to another or have resigned themselves to an unsatisfying relationship. Co-dependents *can* have happy and healthy relationships.

This book is for co-dependent couples who are ready to break out of the painful cycle of dysfunction, to learn how to have healthy intimacy with each other. Although this book is directed to couples who already have a committed sexual relationship, couples just starting out together will also find this book useful.

Many frustrated co-dependent couples make the tragic mistake of ending their relationship before the miracle of recovery has a chance to heal it. Although some relationships do need to end, many are salvageable. Our entrance into recovery from co-dependence does not automatically indicate that we should end our relationship. That's like

"throwing out the baby with the bath water." Couples
who have invested time and effort in their relationships,
but have not been able to make them work, can learn to
heal and grow together.

Before I proceed further, it is important to define some
of the terms I will be using in the chapters that follow. In
the past few years these new terms have almost become
household words to the American public. The terms,
"Adult Children of Alcoholics," "Adult Children of Dysfunctional Families," "Co-dependence" and "The Co-dependent Relationship" are all defined below. Each of these
terms is an attempt to describe a person from a dysfunctional background and their behavioral characteristics.
The term "Recovering Couple" is also defined as it is used
throughout the book. I hope that soon recovering couples
will become as commonplace as unhappy co-dependent
couples currently seem to be.

For the purposes of this book, the following broad
definitions apply:

Adult Children of Alcoholics: People raised in a
family where a parent, grandparent or other family
member was an alcoholic.

Adult Children of Dysfunctional Families: People
from family systems that were consistently unable to
provide a safe nurturing environment. Some examples
of dysfunctional families are those in which there is
physical abuse, emotional abuse, sexual abuse or an
untreated addiction (such as chemical dependence).

Co-dependent: A person raised in a dysfunctional
family who is emotionally dependent on an outside
source to get feelings of self-esteem. The co-dependent focuses on external stimuli in order not to
feel their own pain.

Co-dependent Relationship: A co-dependent in a relationship with another co-dependent or with a person whose behavior is out of control (such as an
alcoholic or other person with a compulsive addictive
disease).

Recovering Couple: Partners in a relationship who are committed to each other and to seeking recovery from their co-dependency. This couple uses their relationship as a vehicle for the transformation from dysfunction to health.

The common thread that ties all these terms together is that all involve adult children who come from dysfunctional family systems. The adult child of an alcoholic is from a dysfunctional family, so is the co-dependent. Co-dependence is the direct result of being raised in any kind of dysfunctional family. All such families develop the same general set of family rules to live by and teach these rules of dysfunction to their children. Adult children bring these rules into their adult sexual relationships, thereby continuing the same dysfunctional patterns. Throughout this book I use the term "co-dependent" to describe adult children from all types of dysfunctional families.

The models and case histories, used here to explain patterns of dysfunctional behaviors, evolved directly from my clinical work with co-dependents. Based on my experience, I believe that the dysfunctional rules and unhealthy patterns of behavior learned in one type of dysfunctional family are much the same in all types of dysfunctional families. Consequently, it is also true that, for all co-dependents, recovery from dysfunction follows the same basic process.

Although this book describes the origins of dysfunction, and the unhealthy patterns that exist in co-dependent relationships, equal time is devoted to outlining the process of recovery. Most of the chapters end with an exercise designed to assist partners in actively practicing certain aspects of intimacy and recovery together.

This book is intended as a practical guide for recovering couples seeking to heal the wounds of the past. I am often asked these two questions: "Is it possible to have a healthy relationship?" and, "Is it worth the effort?" My answer to the first question is always a resounding, *"Yes!"* The answer to the second question must come from within the individual. The experience of sharing at a deep level of intimacy with another human being is a wonderful part of the human experience. It does, however, involve risk, commitment, perseverance, humor and love.

Welcome to the work and play of recovering together.

1

Relationships And The Family Of Origin

Growing up in a dysfunctional family system hurts. The co-dependent is an "adult child" who lived through family dysfunction and who, in adulthood, suffers from a wound of the heart that never had a chance to heal. Recovery from co-dependence is the process of healing these childhood wounds. Whether it was healthy or not, the family environment we knew as children has a profound and long-term effect on the relationships we form later as adults. Growing up in a dysfunctional family system, where children's basic needs for personal safety are not met, does make a difference. The more dysfunctional the family of origin, the more difficult it is for its members later on as they attempt to establish and maintain healthy relationships. The co-dependent person's untreated childhood wounds prevent them from enjoying a relaxed intimacy in any of their relationships, but often they feel the most devastating effects of co-dependence in sexual relationships.

1

All co-dependents have difficulty in sexual relationships because their first role models regarding sexual intimacy (generally parents) were dysfunctional. The pain co-dependents feel in relationships springs from a conflict between their natural desire to bond intimately with another human being and their familiar patterns of dysfunctional behavior. It is important that each partner in an intimate relationship learn about and understand their individual family of origin. With this knowledge they can begin to break the unhealthy patterns that inhibit, even sabotage, their efforts to enjoy a loving closeness to another person.

During a group counseling session a co-dependent named Jan asked, "What is a healthy relationship?" She answered her own question by saying, "I sure don't know! The only role models I had were my parents. My dad was drunk most of the time, and my mother constantly bitched at him. I never saw them hug each other or be affectionate. In my relationships I make guesses at what's healthy. And I think most of the time I guess wrong."

Jan's lack of knowledge about a healthy relationship is typical of most co-dependents. Her frame of reference for relationships was her family of origin, an alcoholic family. The alcoholic family is only one of many different kinds of dysfunctional family systems.

What Is A Dysfunctional Family?

A *dysfunctional family* is one that is consistently unable to provide a safe nurturing environment. Through its maladaptive behaviors, this family develops a set of restrictions that inhibit the social and emotional growth of its members, particularly the children. The healthy family, on the other hand, provides safety and nurturing for its members and assists them in their development by setting firm but reasonable limits, rather than imposing rigid constraints.

Co-dependence results from being raised in a dysfunctional family. A person who was raised in dysfunction is always co-dependent and will find themselves in co-dependent relationships. I define a *co-dependent* as someone who is emotionally dependent on an outside source to get feelings of self-esteem and who focuses on external stimuli in order not to feel their own pain. A *co-dependent relationship* forms when a co-dependent person gets into a relationship with another co-dependent or with a person who is out of control (such as an alcoholic or someone with another type of compulsive addictive disease).

What Produces The Dysfunctional Family?

It is important to know that dysfunctional families are unhealthy for a reason. No family consciously makes a decision to become dysfunctional and do harm to its members. Dysfunction stems from a family's desperate attempts to deal with a family member's (or members') disruptive behavior.

Jan's father was an alcoholic: His drinking was out of control. In order to deal with her father's drinking behavior, her family developed ways of coping that would insure that the family would "survive" as a unit. The cost was that the ways of coping became just as harmful to the family members as her father's drinking had been. The alcoholic family is one of the most widely recognized kinds of dysfunctional family systems.

A partial list of other kinds of out-of-control behavior that produce dysfunctional families include:

> drug addiction
> workaholism
> gambling addiction
> eating disorders
> mental disorders
> sexual abuse
> physical abuse
> religious abuse
> emotional abuse

The above list is incomplete. The point is, whenever a family member is out of control, and the rest of the family cannot deal with that member in a healthy way, the family becomes dysfunctional. Adults who have grown up in dysfunctional systems are often called *adult children* because the restrictive character of their family inhibits their emotional growth. As adults, these individuals are forced to respond to adult situations with limited emotional resources. They lack information about healthy living skills due to their unhealthy childhood role models. All people who are raised in dysfunctional families are adult children. It does not seem to matter what type of dysfunctional family the adult child was raised in. All dysfunctional families learn to respond to the out-of-control element in the family with the same set of rigid family rules and similar patterns of behavior.

Ed's family is one example of a non-alcoholic dysfunctional family. When I interviewed Ed for a therapy group, his first statement was, "I don't know where I belong. When I go to adult children of alcoholics (ACoA) meetings, I feel right at home. It's like they're reading my mail and know everything about me! But I'm not from an alcoholic family. No one in my family drinks and I can't find any alcoholism when I search back into my family history." During the interview it came to light that Ed had been physically abused by his father. When Ed was a "bad boy," his father would strip him and beat his bare back and legs with a leather belt, always causing red welts and sometimes causing bleeding. When he beat Ed, his father often quoted, "Spare the rod and spoil the child." Ed clearly came from a dysfunctional family: His father was a child abuser. His mother was co-dependent and did not intervene on Ed's behalf. It is not surprising that Ed felt at home in ACoA meetings even though there was never any drinking in his family. Ed's family adhered to the same four rules that all dysfunctional family systems follow:

1. **Rigidity**
2. **Silence**
3. **Denial**
4. **Isolation**

To one degree or another, every dysfunctional family follows these rules. This is why people from dysfunctional families feel a common bond and an attraction to each other. They are comfortable with others who have learned the same rules, who live their lives according to the same rigid restrictions.

What Is A Healthy Relationship?

When my client, Jan, asked, "What is a healthy relationship?" she was genuinely stumped. She did, however, have a sense that the pain she felt in relationships was the result of not knowing what a healthy relationship would look like. While dysfunctional relationships follow a harsh set of prohibitions, healthy families and relationships have guidelines or ways of being, that are recognizably healthy. These are:

1. **Flexibility**
2. **Expression**
3. **Acceptance**
4. **Intimacy**

To the degree that the above four ways of being exist in a relationship, the relationship can be said to be healthy. No relationship is completely healthy, nor is any relationship completely dysfunctional. The recovery process transforms the rules learned in the dysfunctional family into healthy ways of being.

All couples exist in a *zone of equality*. Each partner in a relationship is at approximately the same level of health or dysfunction. It is unrealistic for one partner in a relationship to view the other partner as either much healthier or much more dysfunctional. Each partner is equal to the other. One partner may appear to have more skills, or to have it "more together" than the other partner, but this is generally an illusion. If one partner were really much healthier than the other, they would probably leave the relationship to seek someone who is closer to their level of health. The "zone of equality" does not imply that each partner is equal in areas such as physical strength, intellectual ability and so on. It does mean that both partners bring to a relationship an equal range of skills and social information.

During group a co-dependent named Carla said, "I don't know why my husband stays with me. He seems so much healthier than I am." Carla continued, "He's very spiritual and never gets angry or loses control. He's always helping other people and everyone who knows him thinks he's a great guy." The group pointed out to Carla that "never getting angry" did not necessarily mean that her husband was particularly "spiritual" or that he was much healthier than Carla. (Later when Carla's husband got into therapy, it turned out that he was repressing a lot of rage he had not known how to express.) Carla's low sense of self-worth led her to believe that her husband was healthier than she was. In reality, Carla and her husband were emotionally equal. Both of them were raised in dysfunctional family systems, both were co-dependent and both were in a co-dependent relationship.

Many people I talk to have asked, "Am I in a co-dependent relationship?" They are usually disappointed and in a relationship that seems to be going nowhere, but are mystified about why it is unhealthy and how it got that way. For a person raised in a dysfunctional family who has not received treatment for their co-dependence, the appropriate question to ask is not, "Am I in a co-dependent relationship?" but rather, "*How dysfunctional* is my co-dependent relationship?"

I designed the Co-dependent Relationship Questionnaire to help answer these questions. The questionnaire can indicate: (1) whether you are currently in a co-dependent sexual relationship; (2) to what degree your current sexual relationship is dysfunctional; (3) whether your past sexual relationships have been co-dependent, and (4) how dysfunctional your past relationships were.

Take some time now to read the instructions and to fill out the questionnaire.

The Co-dependent Relationship Questionnaire

The Co-dependent Relationship Questionnaire can be used to assess whether or not you are in a co-dependent sexual relationship. The questionnaire is most effective if partners answer it separately then review their answers together. If you are not currently in a sexual relationship, answer this questionnaire on the basis of your remembered behavior and feelings during your last relationship. The questionnaire will help you determine whether your previous relationship was co-dependent. Please check the answer below that most closely describes your feelings or behavior. Answer all questions "yes" or "no."

YES   NO

____ ____   1. Do you place your partner's needs ahead of yours?

____ ____   2. Have you ever hit or been hit by your partner?

____ ____   3. Are you afraid to tell your partner when your feelings are hurt?

____ ____   4. Does your partner tell you how to dress?

____ ____   5. Do you smile when you are angry?

____ ____   6. Do you have difficulty establishing personal boundaries and keeping them?

____ ____   7. Is it difficult to express your true feelings to your partner?

____ ____   8. Do you feel nervous and uncomfortable when alone?

____ ____   9. Do you feel rejected when your partner is spending time with friends?

____ ____   10. Is shame what you feel when your partner makes a mistake?

____ ____   11. Do you have sex when you don't want to?

____ ____   12. Do you withhold sex to get even with your partner?

YES   NO

____ ____   13. Do you think your partner's opinion is more important than yours?

____ ____   14. Do you rely on your partner to make most of the decisions in the relationship?

____ ____   15. Do you become very upset when your partner does not follow your plan?

____ ____   16. Are you afraid to let your partner really know what you are feeling?

____ ____   17. Do you keep silent in order to keep the peace?

____ ____   18. Do you feel like you give and give and get little or no return?

____ ____   19. Do you freeze up when in conflict with your partner?

____ ____   20. Are you unhappy with your friendships?

____ ____   21. Do you often find yourself saying, "It's not that bad?"

____ ____   22. Do you feel you are stuck in this relationship?

____ ____   23. Do you have to control your emotions most of the time?

____ ____   24. Do you lose control of your emotions during times of conflict?

____ ____   25. Do you feel that your relationship would fall apart without your constant efforts?

____   Total number of "YES" answers.

Now take a few moments to review your answers. Co-dependent relationships differ in degree of dysfunction, just as dysfunctional families are unhealthy to varying degrees. The higher the number of "yes" answers you have, the more dysfunctional the relationship. The overall score on the questionnaire can help determine the degree of dysfunction. Use the chart below to help you understand your score.

Number of Yes Answers	Degree of Dysfunction
1 to 7	Mildly Dysfunctional
8 to 18	Moderately Dysfunctional
19 to 25	Severely Dysfunctional

If your score was close to the border between two categories, take this into consideration when interpreting your score. For example, if you marked 18 "yes" answers, then your relationship would be moderately to severely dysfunctional. A close examination of each "yes" answer, using the commentary below, will help you understand the intensity of the unhealthy behaviors present in the relationship.

Below is a brief comment on each question. Because each person answers the questionnaire from their own point of view, it is often helpful to go over your answers with a friend or therapist. If you are currently in a sexual relationship, going over each answer with your partner can give both of you information and insight into the relationship. Most relationships have positive aspects. When you examine each of the questions, be aware of and discuss the questions that were answered "no" and acknowledge the positive aspects of the relationship.

YES NO

____ ____ **1. Do you place your partner's needs ahead of yours?**

When one partner in a relationship continually places the other person's needs and wants ahead of their own, the motive is generally not love but a personal sense of low self-esteem. There are times in relationships when it is loving and healthy to place your partner's needs before yours, but if this happens on a frequent basis, it is likely to be dysfunctional behavior. The result is often resentment, and even lower feelings of self-esteem.

___   ___   **2. Have you ever hit or been hit by your partner?**

Physical violence in a relationship is always dysfunctional and destructive. Although the battering of women is the most common type of physical abuse in relationships, a significant number of men are physically abused by their partners. There is also mutual violence in some relationships. No matter who is hitting whom in the relationship, if you answered "yes" to this question, seek professional help.

___   ___   **3. Are you afraid to tell your partner when your feelings are hurt?**

It is impossible for two people to be in a relationship and not at times hurt each other's feelings. The key here is how the feeling of hurt is communicated to your partner. If when your partner hurts your feelings, you smile or just shrug it off and say, "It's no big deal," you are being dishonest. You are being emotionally silent, repressing your true feelings. Most co-dependents, out of a need to survive, learn not to express their feelings. They learn to discount their inner reality. Repeatedly repressing emotions will cause bitterness and anger, and will eventually destroy intimacy in the relationship.

___   ___   **4. Does your partner tell you how to dress?**

When you let your partner make you over into the image he or she wants you to be, this indicates that you don't have a strong sense of self, and are willing to let someone else tell you how you should present yourself to the world. If you constantly seek approval from your partner about how you look, it is most likely because you don't trust your own judgment.

___   ___   **5. Do you smile when you are angry?**

Anger is difficult for most co-dependents to express. In the family of origin children are often punished for showing anger. They are punished by direct physical abuse, withdrawal of affection or both. In the adult relationship this fear of abuse or rejection is the primary cause for difficulty in expressing anger. In many cases the co-dependent in a relationship will smile when saying, "I'm angry at you." This contradiction between the inner emotion and its outer expression discounts the emotional experience of the adult child and confuses the other person in the relationship.

_____ _____ 6. **Do you have difficulty establishing personal boundaries and keeping them?**

The dysfunctional family always emotionally abuses its children and often physically and/or sexually abuses them. When a child is emotionally or physically invaded again and again, the child does not learn to set limits on the behavior of others. For example, a co-dependent who was sexually abused in childhood may either (1) set no limits on their partner's sexual behavior toward them or (2) avoid sexual intimacy altogether. In the co-dependent relationship, both extremes will often be acted out at different times by the same person. This leads to mutual distrust and confusion for both partners.

_____ _____ 7. **Is it difficult to express your true feelings to your partner?**

When a child is denied the right to express real feelings, and instead learns to express only feelings that will gain approval, they will repeat this behavior later in an adult sexual relationship. One common denominator among all co-dependent relationships is the inability to express true feelings. Many adult children have repressed their feelings for so long that they don't know what their true feelings are. They will guess at what they think their partner will approve of and report that feeling, sending mixed messages to their partner. If a person is actually angry, but tells their partner that they are feeling hurt, the partner will be confused. Since the partner is often a co-dependent too, they may not express this feeling of confusion, resulting in misunderstanding and frustration for both people.

_____ _____ **8. Do you feel nervous and uncomfortable when alone?**

A co-dependent focuses on external stimuli to avoid feeling his or her own pain and is emotionally dependent on others for feelings of self-esteem. Alone without distractions, the co-dependent will begin to feel the pain and anger that has been repressed for most of their lives. This can be a frightening experience. Co-dependents also have difficulty being alone because without someone to take care of, they feel worthless. One co-dependent said, "When I am alone, I am with all of my enemies." Many co-dependents try to cover up the pain they feel in isolation by taking care of someone else. This never works, but rather than be alone, the co-dependent will continue to use another person to anesthetize their pain.

_____ _____ **9. Do you feel rejected when your partner is spending time with friends?**

This feeling of rejection stems from the co-dependent's belief that if their partner spends time with others, then they are inadequate and the relationship is doomed. Attempting to be all things to their partner is the co-dependent's way of feeling in control of the relationship. When the partner shows independence by spending time with friends, the co-dependent's feeling of security and control is threatened. The co-dependent then becomes fearful, assuming that the relationship will end if they are no longer needed. If both partners desire healthy intimacy, this cycle of dependency must be broken. The co-dependent must learn that they are valuable and desirable as a whole person, not as a caretaker alone.

_____ _____ **10. Is shame what you feel when your partner makes a mistake?**

Co-dependents take responsibility for their partners' actions and feelings. They feel shame and embarrassment

when their partner makes a mistake because of a belief
that the mistake is a personal reflection on them, rather
than on their partner. They have difficulty separating
their personal identity from their partner's. Taking responsibility for the feelings and actions of one's partner is
an example of unhealthy *blending* in a relationship, indicating an inability to maintain clear personal boundaries.

_____ _____ **11. Do you have sex when you don't want to?**

The expression of love through sex can be one of the
most bonding and intimate aspects of a relationship. But
sex without clear personal limits can be abusive and degrading. Almost all co-dependents have confusion about
where to set sexual limits. Having sex when you don't
want to, because you think you have to or because you
are afraid to say, "No, not right now" is degrading. Being
forced to have sex against your will is abusive and is no
different than being physically assaulted and beaten up.

_____ _____ **12. Do you withhold sex to get even with
your partner?**

Using sex to get even with your partner for something
they did that you didn't like, or using sex to get your way
almost always backfires and is very damaging to the
relationship. Unfortunately many co-dependents learned
this behavior long ago by watching their parents. Co-
dependents who use sex as a weapon may believe that
this is the only real power they have.

_____ _____ **13. Do you think your partner's opinion is
more important than yours?**

In a healthy relationship both partners' opinions have
equal importance. This is not so in the co-dependent
relationship. Co-dependents learned as children that their
opinions did not matter. Some learned that it could even
be dangerous to express an opinion. Consequently, they
have a deep sense of uncertainty about their ability to
make good choices. They believe that their partner is

better qualified, smarter and more capable of making good decisions. This idea is often encouraged by their partner, who may take advantage of their indecisiveness to control what happens in the relationship.

_____ _____ **14. Do you rely on your partner to make most of the decisions in the relationship?**

One major co-dependent characteristic is an unwillingness to take responsibility for one's own decisions and actions. One or both partners may be so unwilling to make decisions that they will continue to put off decisions until they are decided by default. One partner may evade making decisions until the other partner is forced to make the choice. The fear of making decisions often has its roots in fear of making the wrong choice and being shamed and ridiculed as a result.

_____ _____ **15. Do you become very upset when your partner does not follow your plan?**

The need to control is an important component of the co-dependent's defense system. Co-dependents feel safe when they plan ahead and often feel threatened when their plan is not followed. The reason co-dependents feel safe when they are in control and rigidly following a plan (generally of their own design) is directly related to their growing up in a dysfunctional family system. The dysfunctional family revolves around an element (an alcoholic, for instance) that is out of control and often dangerous. The co-dependent views control and rigidity in a relationship as desirable and safe. When their partner either changes plans or is unwilling to follow their plan, the co-dependent experiences loss of control and becomes afraid.

_____ _____ **16. Are you afraid to let your partner really know what you are feeling?**

This fear is directly related to one of the messages parents in dysfunctional families communicate to their children — that certain feelings are unacceptable and if you display or talk about these forbidden feelings, you are a bad person who will be rejected or shamed by the family. In adult relationships the co-dependent responds to this parental message by hiding these emotions in the belief that if their partner really knew what they were feeling, they would be rejected.

___ ___ **17. Do you keep silent in order to keep the peace?**

Fear of rocking the boat is common to many co-dependents. In childhood they learned it was unsafe to speak out and draw attention to themselves. Co-dependents learned it was not acceptable to talk about what they felt and saw. Some learned by watching their mother and father rage at each other that conflict could be dangerous. When these people grow up and get into co-dependent relationships, they are afraid to challenge their partner, to ask for what they want or to express their true feelings. They try to keep the peace at all costs.

___ ___ **18. Do you feel like you give and give and get little or no return?**

Within the co-dependent relationship one of the partners will frequently give away their personal power, or the ability to take action in one's own behalf. The partner who continually gives, placing their own wants and needs last, eventually feels frustrated and resentful. Because the cause of this frustration and resentment often goes unrecognized, the giving partner may feel swallowed up by the relationship. In fact, the pattern of compulsive giving itself prevents the giver from getting their needs met in the relationship.

___ ___ **19. Do you freeze up when in conflict with your partner?**

Many co-dependents had violent childhoods, and learned to survive family violence by becoming emotionally numb and mentally blank. This state is often described by co-dependents as *freezing up*. In the adult relationship, co-dependents freeze up when they are in conflict with their partner. Even though there may be no threat of violence in the conflict situation, the co-dependent will respond as if violence were about to occur. The freezing up response makes it very difficult to resolve conflict, which naturally occurs in all relationships.

____ ____ **20. Are you unhappy with your friendships?**

When co-dependents get into a relationship, they tend to focus their complete attention on their partner and drop their friends. They try to get all their needs met by one person, their partner. Of course, this is impossible and places a lot of stress on the relationship. Some co-dependents take on their partner's friends and do not keep contact with friends of their own. While it is both desirable and healthy to have mutual friends in a relationship, it is also important for each partner to have personal friends they can talk to and get support from. If each partner does not have the positive support of close friends, the relationship becomes confining. It is also important for the adult child to select the right kinds of friends. Recovery involves finding friends who are positive and supportive rather than critical and negative.

____ ____ **21. Do you often find yourself saying, "It's not that bad?"**

Denial is one of the many ways that co-dependents stay in unhealthy relationships. They repeatedly make excuses for intolerable behavior on the part of their partner and then try to talk themselves into believing that everything is okay. "We hardly talk to each other, but it's not that bad," or "Sometimes when he loses his temper, he hits me but not that hard." These excuses are a part of the denial that co-dependents use to cover up the pain of being in an unhealthy relationship. If you find yourself saying, "It's not that bad," then ask yourself, "How bad does it have to get?"

_____   _____   **22. Do you feel you are stuck in this relationship?**

The feeling of being stuck in a relationship is related to the belief by the co-dependent that this is the last chance they will ever have for a relationship. Co-dependents have experienced so many losses in childhood they feel unable to tolerate one more and desperately cling to their partner. They feel choiceless. It's this relationship or none. Since the relationship is co-dependent and basically unhealthy, there is also a feeling of wanting to escape. The co-dependent's desire to be free of an unhealthy situation, coupled with the fear of losing the relationship, results in the sense of being stuck. This trapped feeling is often one of the first steps in the co-dependent's recovery process.

_____   _____   **23. Do you have to control your emotions most of the time?**

Children raised in dysfunctional families learn that showing certain emotions is not acceptable. They learn that if they show these unsafe emotions, they will be punished — either physically beaten or shamed and ostracized. Anger, hurt and fear are most often repressed. When these children grow up and enter into co-dependent relationships, they bring with them a need (based in fear) to control their emotions. Keeping rigid control over emotional experience in a relationship prevents co-dependents from becoming intimate with a partner. Being capable of emotional vulnerability (trust) is one of the foundations of a healthy sexual relationship.

_____   _____   **24. Do you lose control of your emotions during times of conflict?**

Most co-dependents do not know how to deal with conflict in relationships. Their view is that conflict is bad and dangerous. They may have seen their parents deal with conflict by fighting, yelling, hitting and other violent behavior, or watched their parents meet conflict with silent contempt and blame. In either case, the co-dependent

developed strong, and sometimes overwhelming feelings
surrounding conflict situations. When conflict happens in
the adult relationship, the co-dependent may lose control
in the form of rage or deep sobbing and crying. The co-
dependent then often feels shame and guilt for the emotional outburst, thus adding more tension to an already
heavily charged situation.

_____ _____ **25. Do you feel that your relationship would
fall apart without your constant efforts?**

In the co-dependent relationship there is often one
partner who takes on the responsibility of keeping the
relationship together. This partner is always trying to
smooth over conflict and make things right in the relationship. These people feel as though the relationship is
a great weight on their shoulders, but they are compul-
sively committed to making it work. The harder they
work, however, the more distant and uncooperative their
partner usually becomes. They are caught in a down-
ward cycle of working harder and harder as the relationship gets more and more unhealthy.

After you have completed the questionnaire and have
discussed the answers and comments with your partner,
you both will probably have discovered some interesting
new information about your relationship. Do not be discouraged if you have a lot of "yes" answers. The questionnaire was designed to indicate where in the relationship improvement must take place, not to judge whether
or not the relationship is hopeless. Being willing to do the
questionnaire, and to discuss it is evidence that you both
have begun the process of healing and recovery together.

2

The Rules Of
Family Dysfunction

"Why am I always getting into relationships with women who hurt me?" John asked this question during a co-dependent therapy group session. He continued, "It seems that when I go into a room filled with people, I will zero in on the one woman who will hurt me the most." The men and women in the group nodded their heads in agreement. Each person replied that they had had the same experience.

John's question is one of the most common asked by co-dependents. They want to know why they get into, and stay in, painful and unhealthy relationships. The answer is simple. They are attracted to others who learned in childhood to follow the same narrow restrictions that they themselves learned.

People from dysfunctional families are attracted to each other because they share a common way of living in the world. They share the silent language of dysfunction in the form of strict behavioral rules. I have heard it said that dysfunctional families do not communicate with each other. On the contrary, they do communicate but in silence. Dysfunctional families are masters of indirect communication, so that their children reach adulthood knowing only how to communicate "sideways." When a co-dependent meets another co-dependent, both immediately recognize in each other the behaviors so familiar to them from their upbringing. A co-dependent relationship forms around a nonverbal agreement that both partners will continue to follow these rules of dysfunction. Both partners seek comfort by recreating together the illusion of control and predictability inherent in these rules. Living according to the old family rules is not a choice for co-dependents. As children, they were forced to live by these family rules as a matter of emotional and sometimes physical, survival. This is why the co-dependent person comes to feel that the rigid controls learned in childhood are not only comfortable and familiar but absolutely essential. It is no wonder that co-dependents gravitate toward others who feel as firmly attached to these restrictions as they do. They feel that if they let go of the rules, they might not live through it.

Co-dependents do survive changing their dysfunctional patterns but we'll talk about what it takes to recover a little later on. Right now, though, let's look at the dysfunctional rules themselves.

Remember that these rules are not created in a vacuum. A desperate family turns to this set of rigid behaviors in order to combat the pain of the constant chaos they live with. But however useful they are in times of crisis, these rules sabotage all possibility of intimacy with others in the long run. Here is a brief discussion of the four rules of the dysfunctional family (Rigidity, Silence, Denial and Isolation) and how they affect sexual relationships.

Rigidity

Rigidity is the beginning of dysfunction in a family. When a family member's actions are unpredictable and even dangerous to others, the family will try to rigidly control behavior and emotional expression in an attempt to bring back a sense of order to the family system. Rules are made, never to be broken, and the behavior of all family members is thus expected to be predictable. If one family member deviates from these rigid expectations, the rest of the family will punish them by shaming, ignoring and even physically abusing them. For the dysfunctional family, rigid control is a way to feel safe in an unsafe situation.

In adult relationships the co-dependent attempts to feel safe by applying rigid expectations to the behavior and emotional expression of their partner. For the co-dependent, unpredictable behavior (even a healthy spontaneous expression of joy) feels dangerous. When one partner in a co-dependent relationship breaks the rule of rigidity, the other partner feels an exaggerated dread, perceiving a threat to the relationship. In general, when a co-dependent perceives a loss of control, the experience is accompanied by fear. These feelings may not be logical, but they are very intense.

When two co-dependents enter a relationship with each other, both have a need to control the relationship. Sometimes one partner will appear to be the controller in the relationship, when actually the other partner is really doing the controlling. This quiet controller uses silent manipulation and covert actions to sabotage their partner's plans and actions. Frequently the partner who yells loudest about being controlled actually dominates. No co-dependent relationship escapes control issues because both partners have them and will, in overt and covert ways, fight to control their partner and the relationship. For the co-dependent, the fight for control is a fight for safety — for survival.

Silence

The dysfunctional family imposes the rule of silence on its members to avoid the honest expression of emotions that would reveal its sickness. Rather than expose its shame and despair, the dysfunctional family hides feelings. This is how co-dependents learned to repress their emotional experiences. Fear of losing their parents' love and protection forces co-dependents either to mask their feelings or to deny that they are feeling at all. Many people who are co-dependent shudder at the thought of talking about their true feelings. This barrier of fear is destructive to relationships. Without the honest expression of feelings, intimacy simply cannot happen.

Another aspect of the rule of silence is the fear of talking about what really goes on between family members. Children raised in families that enforce the rule of silence become adults who are unable to talk about behavior that is abusive and unhealthy. They may witness abuse (of themselves or others) but they cannot acknowledge or report it. Co-dependents are also unable to be specific when attempting to ask their partner for what they want (if they ask at all). Co-dependents learned as children to get their needs met by indirect communication and manipulation. As adults, they use suggestions and hints to try to get their partners to give them what they want, rather than asking directly. The rule of silence tells them, "If your partner really loved you, she (or he) would know what you want. You should not have to ask."

Denial

Co-dependents discount their experience of reality, both internally and externally. They may even ignore and minimize behavior that is life-threatening. In the dysfunctional family denial of the problem ("Things aren't that bad") is a way for the family to avoid looking at unhealthy behavior. The family feels safer when everyone acts as if nothing is wrong. Children in the unhealthy system, however, see the unhealthy behavior and feel its effects. They understand something is very definitely wrong, but are told repeatedly that everything is fine. Children also learn by example to pretend not to notice anything that calls attention to the problem, even when it is blatantly obvious. When children are taught that what they see, hear and feel is not real, their ability to trust their own perceptions becomes seriously impaired. The co-dependent's distrust of self is apparent in the extreme anxiety they feel when asked to make decisions based solely on their own observation and intuition.

The co-dependent's habit of discounting reality can keep them in painful and often dangerous situations.

While working as a counselor in a hospital emergency room, I counseled a woman who had been battered by her husband. When I confronted her with the fact that she was being battered, she told me, "It wasn't that bad." I saw this woman for the last time when she was admitted to the emergency room with a gunshot wound to the chest. She died of that wound. She had grown up in a dysfunctional family and had been abused as a child. She married an alcoholic who was a "nice guy" when he was sober but who beat her when he was drunk. This woman's denial was so strong, it kept her from leaving her husband, even to protect her own life.

Denial does not always end in death but it can. Unless denial is acknowledged, the co-dependent person will continue to remain in painful, even dangerous relationships in the belief that "it's not that bad."

Isolation

Essential to intimacy is the ability to be emotionally vulnerable and to make emotional contact. Without this ability, we experience painful isolation from others. Because a dysfunctional family is unable to teach children to express true emotions or to make healthy emotional contact with other family members, the children grow up with a deep feeling of isolation. Regardless of how long a co-dependent stays in a relationship, unless they learn to make emotional contact, their feeling of isolation will persist. Co-dependents sometimes move from relationship to relationship, trying to get rid of their loneliness. Seeking different relationships is futile, though, as long as the co-dependent continues to live by the dysfunctional rules learned in childhood.

The rule of isolation tells the co-dependent not to trust, not to be emotionally vulnerable. Because it was unsafe to be vulnerable as a child, the co-dependent went to great lengths for self-protection. As children they may have been shamed and ridiculed when they displayed unacceptable emotions such as anger, hurt or frustration. As an adult the co-dependent avoids the possibility of humiliation by getting tough, or going numb. Unfortunately, this important survival tool becomes a terrible liability when the co-dependent desires an intimate relationship (which requires honest sharing).

The belief that others cannot be trusted leads the co-dependent into an agonizing predicament. Never having had the nurturance and love that is essential to all people, the co-dependent wants more than anything to feel intimate with another. Having been shamed and punished for showing their true thoughts and feelings, the co-dependent's worst fear is trusting another person enough to experience that intimacy. One client described this conflict well when she remarked, "I desperately wanted to be intimate. At the same time, I was afraid of being intimate. It was very painful and confusing."

The rules of the dysfunctional family exist in the life of every co-dependent. How intensely we experience the rules will depend on how dysfunctional our family was. In general the more dysfunctional the family of origin, the greater effect the rules will have on our relationships. Some people have more difficulty with some rules than with others, and some experience all the rules to about the same degree. Whatever the case, the rules of dysfunction will be transformed by the process of recovery. Facing old patterns of rigidity, silence, denial and isolation is a way to begin to heal.

The Joint Family Tree

To get a clearer idea of the individual family history that both partners bring to a relationship, it is helpful to do a *Joint Family Tree*, a genealogy chart combining both partners' families of origin. A Joint Family Tree creates a dramatic visual representation of the roots of family dysfunction for both partners.

When making your family trees, you may find that your information or memory about some of your family members is incomplete. This is an indication of the silence that is common in dysfunctional families. Work with the information you have, rather than worry about what is missing.

Trace your joint family history back to both sets of grandparents. This will show your parents' (and your partner's parents') families of origin. At the end of this chapter is the Joint Family Tree of Jack and Mary, who have been married for seven years. Use their tree as a model to create your own. You'll see that Jack is represented by the triangle at the lower right of the page and Mary is represented by the circle at the lower left of the page. Their current ages are written in the circle and triangle. The length of time they have been married is written on a line connecting "Jack" and "Mary."

Moving upward on the page, "Mary" is connected by a line drawn to her parents' names, "Harry" and "Judy." Mary's name is placed in the correct birth order between her sisters' and brother's names. Mary's father died at the age of 65 so his triangle is marked with an "X," indicating that he is deceased. The same format is repeated for both of Mary's parents, completing Mary's family tree as far as her grandparents. John has completed his own family tree in the same way. Once they had completed their Joint Family Tree, Jack and Mary added any dysfunctional behavior or disease that was applicable ("workaholic," "alcoholic" or "co-dependent") next to the names of certain family members. Follow the same format as you construct your own Joint Family Tree. When you have each completed your half of the chart, share with your partner how it felt to do this. Below are several open-ended statements designed to facilitate discussion. Each partner is to complete each of the statements.

1. What I learned about my family was. . . .
2. What I learned about your family was. . . .
3. I was surprised by. . . .
4. After doing this Joint Family Tree, I feel. . . .

As you both find more information about your respective families, continue to update and revise the Joint Family Tree. Review the chart occasionally and discuss whether your feelings about your family and your partner's family, have changed. Continue to review how your respective families of origin have had an impact on your relationship with each other.

Figure 2.1. Joint Family Tree

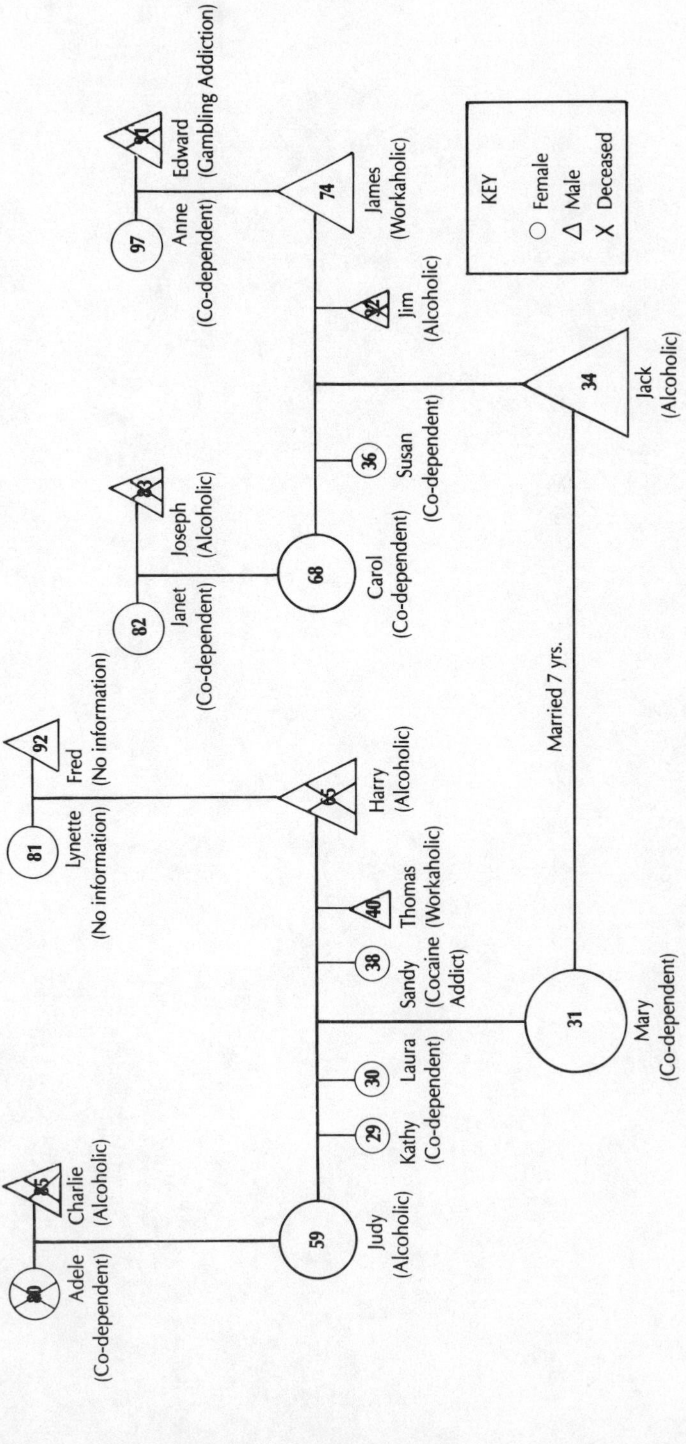
Adele
(Co-dependent)
Charlie
(Alcoholic)
Lynette
(No information)
81
Fred
(No information)
92
Janet
(Co-dependent)
82
Joseph
(Alcoholic)
Anne
(Co-dependent)
97
Edward
(Gambling Addiction)
Judy
(Alcoholic)
59
Kathy
(Co-dependent)
29
Laura
(Co-dependent)
30
Sandy
(Cocaine
Addict)
38
Thomas
(Workaholic)
40
Harry
(Alcoholic)
Carol
(Co-dependent)
68
Susan
(Co-dependent)
36
Jim
(Alcoholic)
James
(Workaholic)
74
Married 7 yrs.
Mary
(Co-dependent)
31
Jack
(Alcoholic)
34
KEY
○ Female
△ Male
X Deceased

3

New Ways Of Being

Recovery from the dysfunctional family rules and from the issues of abandonment and engulfment is a lifelong process. Recovery is not an event; it is a healthy way of being in the world. Recovering through relationships is dynamic and ever-changing. A co-dependent named Mike summed up his feelings about recovery this way: "I desperately wanted to hurry my recovery so I could 'graduate.' Then I wouldn't have to do any more work; I would be all well and finished. When I realized that wasn't going to happen, I was depressed. Then I learned that recovery really is a *process*. I don't have to do it perfectly and I don't have to rush things. I have the rest of my life to get healthier and healthier. What a relief!" Mike's insights were important information for him. He realized that recovery was not a race to the finish line. Instead Mike's recovery had become an interesting journey that led to healthier and more satisfying ways of living.

It is important to remember that recovery is an individual commitment. The choice to recover must be made by

the individual who wants a change. It cannot be forced
upon anyone. At the same time none of us enters recovery
in isolation. Recovery from a dysfunctional family means
learning how to be healthy in all human relationships —
with friends, co-workers, children, parents, siblings, but
especially with our life partner.

We have seen that the families of co-dependents teach
and enforce dysfunctional rules on their children. Because
co-dependent people have learned their basic relationship
skills within this maladaptive framework, their recovery
process involves repeatedly breaking each of the dysfunctional family rules. Gradually the old rules evolve into
new healthy ways of being.

The rules of the dysfunctional family are created out of
the desperate need to survive; consequently, they have
tremendous power. Behind each rule is the energy of
survival. Because the dysfunctional rules are basic to the
co-dependent person's feelings of personal safety, it is
impossible just to remove them. Instead, the dysfunctional
behavior must be transformed.

Below are the four rules of dysfunction and the new
ways of being that replace them as recovery deepens:

Rules		Ways of Being
Rigidity ⟶ transformed into ⟶		Flexibility
Silence ⟶ transformed into ⟶		Expression
Denial ⟶ transformed into ⟶		Acceptance
Isolation ⟶ transformed into ⟶		Intimacy

As we have seen, the rules of dysfunction inhibit and
cripple relationships. The "ways of being" enhance and
strengthen intimacy. Let's look at these new ways of being
in more detail.

Flexibility

Partners in any relationship have different, and some-times conflicting, needs and desires. Individual fulfillment is important in a relationship, but if both partners are rigid and inflexible about how this happens, neither of them will feel fulfilled. Instead a core of resentment will grow and will harm the couple's intimacy with each other. Learning to be flexible, to compromise and to negotiate is essential to healthy relationships. Transforming old pat-terns involves letting go of the win-lose atmosphere that characterizes dysfunctional families' interactions with each other. Having the flexibility to work out our differ-ences gives our relationships a sense of harmony and partnership. Nothing makes stern adversaries of a loving couple faster than a rigid refusal to compromise.

Because conflict is natural in every healthy relationship, learning to resolve conflict *as a team* is crucial for couples healing together. Notice how this view considers *the conflict itself as the problem*, rather than placing blame on one partner or the other. If one or both partners are unwilling to compromise or negotiate, conflict goes unresolved. And here is an unsavory fact: Unresolved conflict will always arise again later, usually with more force than it had to begin with. Healthy couples sometimes have to "agree to disagree," which is still preferable to an angry stalemate in which neither partner can tolerate a view-point that differs from their own.

Margaret entered therapy to learn how to improve her current relationship. Like many co-dependent people, she had great difficulty learning to negotiate with her lover. Her attitude was, "I know when I'm right, and I know what I want. Why should I negotiate?" Margaret had learned from her parents that in every conflict one person "won" and the other "lost." There was no middle ground. Whoever lost the battle would then plot to get even or try to get what they wanted by using manipulation. In Margaret's family of origin winning an argument was one of the few ways she could feel good about herself. It meant she was better and stronger than the "loser." But this short-term self-esteem was costly for Margaret. Time after time her relationships had ended in anger and disappointment. Margaret did not know how to be flexible. In order to coexist peacefully and happily with her lover, she had to learn to let go of control and become less rigid. Breaking the rule of rigidity always involves releasing control, a scary prospect for co-dependents. But the reward of learning to negotiate and compromise is to enjoy real friendship with our life partner. Flexibility and tolerance allow recovering couples freedom from the destructive effort to control that exists in dysfunctional relationships. When change, adjustment and flexibility are understood as necessary to loving another person, partners are free to take risks with each other, to be creative and spontaneous. Flexible couples allow for each other's human shortcomings. Rather than gloat over errors and regrets, healthy partners extend support to each other through their willingness to adapt.

Expression

The cold and confusing silence of dysfunctional families creates miscommunication, misunderstanding and resentment. Expression creates openness and builds intimacy in a relationship. To speak openly about what we feel, hear and see (discussing difficult feelings as well as voicing appreciation) is to act with integrity. The practice of honest expression contradicts everything the co-dependent was taught to believe about communication.

Relationships are full of deep feelings. Co-dependent people experience fears of abandonment and engulfment and even the happiest couples feel angry and hurt with each other at times. For some, jealousy is a problem. Whatever the emotions, nothing damages trust more surely than failing to express them. For a couple to experience together the special connectedness that is the earmark of a healthy relationship, risk is necessary. Great courage is required for co-dependents to honestly vent their feelings. They fear that their partner will reject or ridicule their emotions, having experienced this again and again as children. (Of course, if our partner has been abusive and discounting in the past, we have reason to expect that they will respond with rejection or ridicule again.) Taking the risk to be vulnerable by expressing feelings to a *trustworthy* partner is an important step in breaking the cycle of silence.

During a group session one woman voiced a fear common to most co-dependents. Joan told the group, "I'm afraid to tell my husband when I'm angry at him. I'm afraid he'll go away and never come back if I get as mad as I really feel." Joan was acting on her childhood training. When she had shown anger as a child, her father had punished her by walking away and refusing to speak to her based on his belief that "good little girls don't get angry." In reality everyone gets angry sometimes, including "good little girls." Part of being human means feeling a *complete range* of emotions. Labeling some emotions "acceptable" and others "unacceptable" robs children of their birthright, to be fully human.

In addition to honestly expressing feelings, it is important to ask our partner for what we want from them. Many co-dependents rarely express their wishes because they have learned always to consider others' needs before their own. As children, co-dependents were told their needs were unimportant. Or they were taught that making requests was selfish or immoral. Co-dependents often wish that their partners were mind-readers. They would not have to ask for what they wanted because their partner would somehow just know what it was. For this reason we co-dependents have spent a lot of time in relationships feeling disappointed and resentful, complaining that our partner is not giving enough to us. In reality if we want something from our partner, we must express our desire for it. This is risky because revealing our desires tells a lot about who we are. And there's the risk that our partner will not do what we've asked. But this is an outcome we can learn to live with. Recovery sometimes

means just feeling disappointed, without resorting to unhealthy methods of "getting our way." What's most important is our *willingness to ask* for our needs to be met, rather
than wait for our loved ones to guess what we want. We
may need something as easy to request as a quiet hour to
ourselves or as difficult to ask for as a different kind of
sexual touch. But we must ask if our partner is to have
the opportunity to give.

Marty, a co-dependent, once shared this story about
asking for what you want: "I wouldn't ask my wife for
what I wanted when we made love, so she would guess.
When Anna guessed wrong, I would be angry at her for
not meeting my needs. Then *she* would get angry and
hurt because I was angry at *her*. Then I would get even
angrier that she didn't understand me. It just became a
crazy cycle. When I learned to ask Anna for what I
wanted, things got much better between us. I didn't always get what I asked for, but she knew what I wanted
and that stopped the cycle of hurt and resentment."

Breaking the silence by expressing feelings is risky.
There's always the possibility that we won't like our
partner's response. But healthy risk-taking is essential for
the recovering couple to develop that famous prerequisite
to intimacy: trust.

Acceptance

Regarding these new ways of being in healthy relationships, two kinds of acceptance are important to consider.
The first is acceptance of yourself, exactly as you are
right now, and the second is acceptance of your partner
exactly as they are right now.

Because children raised in dysfunctional families are
pressured to deny reality, they inherit two damaging lies.
As "adult children," they carry in their hearts the mistaken belief that (1) there is nothing wrong with their
family of origin, and (2) something is basically deeply
wrong at the very core of themselves. They accept other
people's (usually their parents') ideas about what they

should be feeling and thinking. Early on, at a deep level, co-dependents learn not to accept themselves.

One of the first steps in self-acceptance is to begin accepting that our feelings are real, and that it is all right to express them. When clients tell me, "I don't know what I feel," I know they are genuinely confused, that they have been trained to hide or redirect their emotions.

A client named Greg was used to redirecting his feelings. He came into therapy because he was tired of being angry all the time. During group he revealed that as a boy, he was told that it was unmanly to show fear or to cry. But by watching his father's angry explosions, Greg had learned that anger was acceptable to express. Since showing pain or fear was unacceptable, Greg also showed anger even when he was feeling hurt or afraid. He learned to redirect his emotions so well that by the time he entered therapy, he was entirely unable to recognize when he felt pain or fear. He had mistakenly concluded that he just did not experience those emotions. During the course of therapy, Greg learned to recognize that he often feared abandonment and that he felt hurt about having been expected to act like an adult when he was a small child. To feel good about himself as a whole person, Greg had to accept all of his emotions, not just those his parents had accepted.

Once we accept ourselves as we are, accepting our partner becomes much easier to do. Many co-dependents fall in love with a fantasy about the kind of person their partner might become, and do not learn much about who their partner really is. Because they are in love with a dream, they become frustrated whenever their partner's behavior does not match the fantasy. They feel determined to change their partner to fit this dream. This situation is not love at all and, what's more, it can never work. Imperfect human beings just cannot live up to dreams and fantasies in which everything is perfect (unreal, perhaps, but perfect!). Accepting our partner, with their shortcomings as well as their endearing qualities, makes for a much more realistic and meaningful relationship. Loving the human being rather than the fantasy brings to the relationship respect and dignity: two signs of genuine love.

Elena, a client in group therapy, said this about letting go of her fantasy husband: "When I stopped trying to love what I *wanted* my husband to be, and tried just to love *him*, I found out that I really didn't love him at all. We broke up. In my current relationship with Mike, I really looked at him closely, to really know him before I got involved with him. I try not to change him. I feel better about myself, too, and things are going much better this time."

Notice that Elena mentioned that she felt better about *herself*. Once again, regarding ourselves as worthwhile is essential to a loving and healthy bond with our partner. This is important to remember because acceptance of our partner never means accepting abusive behavior. We do not have to accept behavior that is dangerous or abusive, either physically or emotionally. Acceptance does not involve continually putting ourselves at risk. Rather, it is the gentle art of loving ourselves as we are and supporting our partner in loving themselves as well. True acceptance often brings about positive changes in a relationship.

Intimacy

The depth and richness of a healthy sexual relationship comes from *intimacy*: a satisfying sense of sharing oneself that, to the co-dependent, feels foreign. Most co-dependents do not experience intimacy in their sexual relationships. As we have seen, dysfunctional families teach rules which prevent intimacy. A relationship without intimacy has an empty spot in the middle of it — compared to a healthy partnership, it is not much of a relationship at all. Though co-dependents may use various means to erase their persistent feelings of isolation and emptiness in relationships, nothing can fill up that emptiness except breaking the rules of dysfunction in order to build real intimacy together.

Co-dependents usually believe that love and intimacy go hand and hand — that if two people fall in love, intimacy always follows. This is false. Mystical and magical though it is, the extraordinary experience we have named "falling in love" *by itself* is not enough to maintain a healthy committed relationship between two people. Falling in love makes us feel as if we are as warmly close to our lover as is humanly possible. But partners must learn the art (and work) of intimacy as well, if the relationship is to continue in a healthy way.

Intimacy in the sexual relationship occurs naturally when both partners are able to risk sharing their feelings and to remain in the relationship when conflict (inevitably) arises. When we trust ourselves and our partners enough to ask for our needs to be met, when we are willing to negotiate and compromise, then intimacy happens spontaneously.

Intimacy is the ability not only to physically touch our partner in tender and exciting ways, but to profoundly contact their essential self (who they really are) on a consistent basis.

Ralph, a co-dependent in group therapy, stated he had believed at one time that being intimate meant having sex. Ralph reported, "I always liked having sex. It was exciting and fun. After a while, though, I would start to feel emotionally empty, like there was a hole in my heart. Then I'd go out and find a different lover, and that emptiness would go away for a little while. But sooner or later the feeling always came back and the cycle would start all over again. When I learned to risk talking about my feelings and staying in this relationship with Barb — really making a commitment to work things out — the emptiness began to disappear."

There are four dimensions of intimacy in a relationship: physical, emotional, mental and spiritual. For co-dependent partners to heal together, they must consciously open themselves to all four dimensions.

Summary

The transformation from the dysfunctional rules of the unhealthy family system into healthy ways of being is an ongoing process. Co-dependents learned the rules of Rigidity, Silence, Denial and Isolation over a long period of time. These unhealthy patterns will not disappear in a day or a week. Recovery is the process of breaking and transforming the rules of dysfunction again and again until healthy behavior comes naturally. It is a long process but the results of opening ourselves to this transformation are extraordinary. We experience the benefits of our efforts very quickly. Living the new ways of being — Flexibility, Expression, Acceptance and Intimacy — is an exciting and rewarding experience. Each one of us deserves it! In the next chapter are some concrete suggestions and strategies for entering this important transformation.

Talking About Feelings: An Exercise

Since most co-dependents have difficulty identifying and expressing feelings, it is helpful for the recovering couple to consciously practice identifying feeling states. Below is a list of open-ended statements about feelings. Using this list can help you become more comfortable talking with your partner about feelings. Practicing this kind of communication is one way to deepen the bond you have with each other.

Here are some guidelines:

Take turns being first to complete the statements.
Try to respond to each statement before going on to the next.
Either partner may decline to complete any statement.
Either partner may end the session at any time.

1. I feel happy when . . .
2. I feel sad when . . .
3. I feel affectionate when . . .
4. I feel hurt when . . .
5. I feel loving when . . .
6. I feel shy when . . .
7. I feel excited when . . .
8. I feel anxious when . . .
9. I feel joyful when . . .
10. I feel ashamed when . . .
11. I feel angry when . . .
12. I feel confused when . . .
13. I feel playful when . . .
14. I feel frustrated when . . .
15. I feel blissful when . . .
16. I feel jealous when . . .
17. I feel secure when . . .
18. I feel worried when . . .
19. I feel delighted when . . .
20. I feel resentful when . . .
21. I feel hopeful when . . .

22. I feel grief when . . .
23. I feel loss when . . .
24. I feel exhilarated when . . .
25. I feel embarrassed when . . .
26. I feel afraid when . . .
27. I feel tender when . . .
28. I feel desperate when . . .
29. I feel peaceful when . . .
30. I feel loved when . . .

This is only a partial list of feeling states. Add your own feeling statements to this list. You might try using a thesaurus, or book of synonyms, to find other words to describe nuances of emotional expression. With your partner, make a game of using different words to describe feeling states throughout the day. You may be surprised to find out how many different kinds of emotions you really feel.

4

Elements Of Recovery

Having read about the four rules of the dysfunctional family and the four ways of being, you may be asking, "How can my relationship make the transformation from the Rules of Dysfunction to the Ways of Being?" The impulse behind this question is accurate. Just knowing that change is necessary is not enough. It's like going to a banquet and not being able to taste the food. Looking at delicious food whets the appetite, but it does nothing to take away the hunger; it only makes us more eager to taste what we have seen. The co-dependent couple must create a plan of action in order to bring recovery into their relationship. Then they can proceed past the stage of knowing that their way of relating is unhealthy and unsatisfying and on to developing healthy ways of being together. The four Elements of Recovery (below) are necessary to bridge the gap between dysfunctional and healthy behavior:

Behavioral Action   **Cognitive Reconstruction**
Emotional Expression   **Spiritual Awareness**

The four Elements of Recovery reflect the natural planes of existence that contain all human experience: physical, emotional, mental and spiritual. Because all dysfunctional families have some combination of physical abuse, sexual abuse and emotional abuse, as well as abandonment and engulfment (see Chapter 6), co-dependents have sustained damage on each of these four planes. Conscious work in *each* of these areas is necessary for *full and meaningful* recovery to take place in the co-dependent relationship. Now we'll look at each of the elements of recovery and the part they play in healing your relationship to your partner.

Behavioral Action

Behavioral action means taking action to change old behavior. It may sound simple, but it isn't. For co-dependent people, letting go of the old familiar behavior they learned in childhood means moving into uncomfortable, unfamiliar territory.

I heard a joke once about co-dependence that goes: "A co-dependent is someone who gets into a rut, and then moves in furniture." The joke is funny because there is a ring of truth in it. The co-dependent will continue to behave in the same unhealthy ways because the old habits are comfortable and make life seem more manageable (for a while, at least). Unfortunately some co-dependents' fear of change is greater than the pain it causes them to stay in the rut of disappointing relationships.

Changing behavior means that the co-dependent must act, not only in the face of intense feelings of fear, but also in the face of the old myth that "This will never work." Co-dependents have an inner commentator (the internalized voice of their dysfunctional family) always telling them to wait before making a change: "Wait until there is no fear or pain involved," this voice advises. The problem is that if the co-dependent waits until there is no fear or pain involved, they will probably stay stuck forever. It is the change in behavior that decreases the pain and fear. These feelings will not go away by themselves.

Ellen, a co-dependent, was in a marriage that was physically abusive. Her husband beat her several times a year.
After each beating, he always swore to her, "I will never
do that again." But sooner or later he would beat her again.
Ellen (who joined one of my therapy groups on the sug-
gestion of friends) felt intense fear whenever she thought
about leaving her husband. She reported thinking to herself, "If I leave him, I will never have another relationship."
As Ellen came to realize how dangerous her situation had
become, she decided that she had to protect herself. With
the support of her therapy group, and her friends, Ellen
acted on her decision by leaving her husband. Even though
she still felt intense fear about being alone, Ellen had to
take behavioral action to ensure her personal safety.

After she had been separated from her husband for
several weeks, Ellen confided in group that the first two
weeks were very hard, that she felt very lonely and really
wanted to go back to her husband. She told us, "I would
sit on my hands so I would not call him." Even though it
caused her emotional pain and fear, Ellen changed her
behavior and continued to practice acting in a healthy
way. After several weeks, Ellen reported that the fear and
loneliness were lessening. She had begun to feel good
about leaving and hopeful about the possibility of having
a healthy relationship in the future. This took place several
years ago and I am happy to report that Ellen is now in
another (much healthier) relationship and has a child.

Behavioral Action means taking healthy action despite
our fear and pain during the change. Sometimes, however,
changing behavior means holding our ground and not
taking any physical action. Some co-dependents leave a
relationship as soon as trouble or conflict occurs, rather
than deal with anger or disagreement. All relationships
have conflict, and it is important to learn that conflict and
fear do not have to end a relationship. For some co-
dependents, staying in a relationship and trying to work
through times of trouble is healthy behavioral change.
They practice taking no action, rather than escape to a
different relationship.

One co-dependent, Dave, said, "As soon as we would get into an argument, I would split. I must have had 10 relationships in the past two years! In all of them I left when things stopped going smoothly. With my fiancee, I'm committed to try to work things out before I ever consider leaving. It's really hard. It's so tempting to run away. But if I don't run, things actually do work out. I'm really amazed!"

Making behavioral changes is important for co-dependents to break out of unhealthy, self-defeating patterns in relationships. Changing behavior is only one part of recovery, however. For complete recovery, the co-dependent must also work with the elements of emotional expression, cognitive reconstruction and spiritual awareness.

Emotional Expression

Healthy *Emotional Expression* is the ability to spontaneously express honest emotions in appropriate ways. The three key words in this definition are "spontaneous," "honest" and "appropriate."

The co-dependent often has difficulty expressing emotions *spontaneously*. Because they have learned not to express certain feelings, they try to completely control their emotional expressions. They do not feel safe expressing what they are feeling at the moment, which makes spontaneity impossible. Co-dependents are often very good at going numb to cover up what they are feeling: As adults, they appear unflappable. Nothing seems to bother them. They are *in control* of their emotions. The price co-dependents pay for this control is the inability to express themselves. They cannot show their joy or their pain. They have a built-in guard against being known by another person. In relationships, some co-dependents show a calm exterior while feeling intense turmoil inside. Such tight control leaves very little room for laughter or play.

Learning to express feelings at the time they are being experienced requires us to trust our partner. Telling our partner, "I was very angry at you," is most helpful if we can say so before a day or a week has passed. Sharing our feelings on the spot speeds the resolution of painful feeling states and unhealthy situations. Unexpressed anger, hurt, grief and other repressed emotions will cause resentments, which can later explode into rage. Repressed emotions always reappear and they do so in many forms. Some of these are explosive rage, inconsolable grief, physical sickness, depression and a wide variety of dysfunctional behaviors.

Many co-dependents are people-pleasers, expressing only what they think others want to hear and see, rather than showing what they really feel. This is not usually *conscious* dishonesty, but it is dishonesty nonetheless. Co-dependents will tell their spouse or lover they feel sad when they are actually angry, or smile when they are hurt. Consequently their partner doesn't really get close enough to know them. In order for a co-dependent relationship to be transformed to a healthy one, each partner must discover where it is that deceit enters into their interactions, to learn to show real feelings rather than masks.

Once a recovering co-dependent develops the ability to risk sharing emotions, a second challenge presents itself: how to respond with real feeling, in the moment, *in an appropriate way*. In the difficult process of change, we may make a great breakthrough by getting angry with our partner but (since we still have only limited role models to draw from) we may shout insults and even break things. The real feelings are showing, but the expression of them is inappropriate. While it is reasonable to expect that we will sometimes make mistakes on our way to learning accurate emotional expression, a lot of damage can come to a relationship if we are not also working on *how* we express our feelings, particularly our anger. Expressing emotions in ways that are abusive to a partner is always damaging to the relationship.

When I interviewed Kim for a co-dependency group, I asked her how she expressed anger. She told me, "I never express anger. As a matter of fact, I don't ever get angry." After several months in group, Kim came to one session looking very tense. When asked what was happening with her, she replied that she was feeling annoyed because she had had a disagreement with her husband. During their disagreement he insulted her and called her a "bitch." The group validated Kim's right to feel annoyed at being insulted and suggested that "annoyed" might be too mild a description to reflect what she was feeling. I have a paddle and a pillow which clients use to express their anger and rage, so I asked Kim to hit the pillow with the paddle while saying, "I'm angry."

When Kim was a child, her mother and father had told her that "good girls didn't get angry." She not only had never learned how to express anger, she had learned to repress her anger altogether. She knew how to express hurt and to cry, but did not know how to get angry. When she began to hit the pillow and say, "I'm angry," she was very uncomfortable. After a few minutes, however, she began to get into the spirit of being angry and began hitting the pillow with a great deal of force and emotion. Kim beat the pillow for almost 40 minutes! During that time she would occasionally look up at the group members and, sweat covering her face, would ask, "Is it really okay to do this? This feels *good*!" She finally stopped because she was too tired to continue. Afterward, Kim reported that she had never felt so free and relaxed.

Kim's case is typical of many co-dependents who have repressed their emotions. After that session Kim was able to go home and tell her husband that she was angry at him. She had begun the process of honestly expressing her emotions.

Learning emotional expression in relationships is vital to the health of the relationship. There can be no true intimacy in a relationship without honest emotional contact between partners.

Cognitive Reconstruction

Cognitive Reconstruction involves using the power of our own minds to replace old unhealthy programming and to learn new relationship skills. We all have the ability to think and to create. We can learn new ideas and unlearn dysfunctional patterns of thought. Co-dependents have a thinking disorder learned from their dysfunctional upbringing. The co-dependent's low self-esteem leads them to believe that they do not deserve to have (or are incapable of having) a happy healthy relationship.

The co-dependent can replace old negative programming with new and healthy attitudes about relationships, by consciously redirecting their thinking. This negative programming comes from the devaluing messages that dysfunctional families give to their children by their actions. Whatever the negative message, the adult co-dependent will act on these self-defeating internal cues unless they learn to interject positive self-encouragement. If our parents gave us the message that, "Sex is dirty and we don't talk about it," this message stays locked in our belief system until a healthy belief replaces it. We can practice replacing that message with "Sex is natural and it's okay to talk about it." Doing this requires a conscious decision on our part. An effective way to practice self-encouragement is the use of affirmations.

Affirmations are healthy thoughts deliberately placed in the mind. When affirmations are repeated over a period of time, they become part of our *recovering* belief system. The affirmations replace the unhealthy messages learned in childhood. Affirmations are most effective when they are short and affirm what is positive (rather than deny what is negative). Using affirmations to change the old, critical messages is extremely helpful in recovery.

Everyone who has been raised in a dysfunctional family is painfully familiar with the phenomenon of having their every action subjected to the running commentary of an internal critic. (Some recovering co-dependents refer to this as "The Committee.") Without practicing cognitive reconstruction, recovery will be limited: The co-dependent will still be left with haunting mental messages like, "You're no good" and, "Your relationships are doomed to fail."

Affirmations will be discussed in greater detail in Chapter 5. For now, here are some examples of affirming statements about healthy relationships:

I am committed to my relationship with _____ .
This relationship is healthy.
I am expressing my true feelings to my partner.
I am happy in my relationship.
My relationship frees me to do what I want to do.

Another aspect of cognitive reconstruction is the ability to solve problems. Many clients have told me, "My best thinking is what got me in trouble." But there is nothing wrong with thinking. Feelings are not all there is to a relationship. What gets co-dependents into trouble is their unhealthy patterns of thinking. They use dysfunctional ideas and beliefs to try to solve their relationship problems.

John, a co-dependent client of mine, thought that the only way to resolve conflict in his marriage was not to talk about problems. He believed that by not talking to his wife about it, the problem would go away. Of course, John's method forced the problem "underground," to reappear at a future time. During therapy John learned that talking about problems actually helped the situation. He was surprised by this discovery, having learned as a child to avoid disagreements at all costs. Now when John senses a problem in the relationship, he thinks about possible solutions and discusses them with his wife.

When two partners apply healthy creative thinking to find solutions to their relationship issues, it is a sure sign of a vital relationship. To solve problems together requires honesty, teamwork and a sharing of our creativity — it means truly giving of ourselves.

Spiritual Awareness

At some point during the recovery process, every co-dependent asks the question, "Why did this happen to me? Why do I have to do all this work just to learn how to have a relationship with someone I love?" Understandably co-dependents want some explanation about why they were born into a family that abused its children. I have never met anyone who found a satisfactory answer to this question without looking into their own beliefs about the very meaning of human existence. The question, "Why?" is often demanding and persistent within co-dependent people and, like repressed feelings, ignoring the need for a spiritual answer will leave a part of recovery unfinished. "Spiritual discontent" often takes the form of a general distrust in the life process and a feeling that the world is not a safe place.

This underlying discontent and distrust affects the co-dependent's relationship in subtle ways. Co-dependents often seek in relationships the spiritual safety that they have been unable to find elsewhere. When one or both persons in a relationship rely on the other to provide spiritual safety and comfort, a great disappointment results. No human being is capable of meeting the spiritual needs of another. Co-dependents who expect always perfect unconditional support and comfort from a human partner are knocking at the wrong address. Imperfect human beings make very poor gods.

Spiritual Awareness means that each partner in a relationship has a spiritual resource that affirms and supports them in the reality of day-to-day living. The couple who share a spiritual practice, religious affiliation or belief system has a resource that will give strength and depth to the relationship.

Years ago I saw a church advertisement on television that said, "The family that prays together stays together." With the arrogance of youth, I ridiculed that concept. Today I believe that this statement is essentially true. Couples need to share a spiritual foundation that can sustain them both when conflict or crisis arises as it does in the best relationships.

In my personal recovery from co-dependence, the awareness of, and reliance on, a Higher Power has given me the freedom to enjoy my marriage. Moving from co-dependence to the co-creation of a healthy family with another loving human being is a joyful experience. The glue that holds it all together is a common belief in a power greater than ourselves, that both I and my partner can call upon for guidance and support in times of need and trouble. There is nothing wrong with relying on and trusting one's partner to provide love and nurturing. Total reliance on another human being, however, is self-sabotage. For a sense of safety in our risk-taking, and for strength through the storms of life, we must look to a spiritual source.

Using the elements of recovery to transform the dysfunctional family rules into healthy ways of being is the essence of the recovery process. Not one of these four elements of recovery, however, can stand alone. Each must be consciously worked on, along with the rest. In this way we experience recovery across the entire range of our experience — we discover what it is to be fully alive in the world.

5

Transformation

There is nothing very mysterious about recovery from co-dependency. It involves specific elements of concrete action. But recovery is by no means easy, and focusing our attention in unproductive ways can lead to frustration and despair. It is easy to get lost and out of balance in the recovery process because it involves so much that is new and unfamiliar to us. A balanced recovery program will include all four of the Elements of Recovery discussed earlier, as well as a lot of perseverance. A common pitfall for co-dependents in recovery is to focus on only one or two of the elements of recovery, excluding the others.

For example, recovery does not go well when we make great effort to practice new ways of thinking about ourselves (cognitive reconstruction) and try new healthy behaviors (behavioral action), if we are neglecting our needs to express our leftover grief and anger (emotional expression), as well as our need for spiritual strength to support us in our risk-taking (spiritual awareness).

Co-dependents who learn only one, two or even three, of these elements will experience limited recovery.

Charlie, a man in his thirties who had been married and divorced four times, had been working on his co-dependency issues for about a year. Through his reading and by talking with other recovering co-dependents, Charlie had learned to change his self-destructive behavior into healthy behavior. Along with the change in his behavior, he had joined a group which taught that affirmations were a way to achieve happiness and personal growth. He also belonged to a spiritual group that taught and practiced spiritual principles. Charlie was involved with three of the four elements of recovery: Behavioral Action, Cognitive Reconstruction and Spiritual Awareness.

Charlie was very enthusiastic about his recovery and said of himself, "I'm much better than I used to be." However, Charlie had entered therapy because he still felt stuck. It soon became apparent that Charlie was stuck in the area of emotional expression. He rarely showed emotions that he believed were negative. He would laugh when he felt happy, but would never reveal his sadness or anger. Even when he was feeling hurt, he would smile and say, "I'm just fine." Charlie's recovery was out of balance. To even out his recovery process, he needed to focus on learning to express all of his emotions. When he began to let himself feel angry, sad and hurt, he felt free and unstuck, so that he could bring his whole emotional self to his relationships.

Unwittingly Charlie had neglected his recovery in the area of emotional expression. Other co-dependents, however, may be emotionally expressive and spiritually aware, but do not take action to change their behavior. There are a variety of ways that the recovery process gets off-center. Looking at all the Elements of Recovery and consciously integrating them into a new program of health assures that our recovery is a balanced process.

Co-dependents should be wary of therapies and therapists claiming to have a single technique that will insure complete recovery. Many therapists are only trained to guide their clients in one or two of the elements of recovery. For example, they may teach and encourage emotional expression (or discharge), but may be unaware of the need for behavioral action, cognitive reconstruction and spiritual awareness.

It is easy to fall into what I call The Therapy Trap. This occurs when a co-dependent (individual or couple) ends up with an untreated co-dependent as their therapist. The therapeutic relationship between the client(s) and therapist is then damaged by the therapist's unresolved co-dependent issues. This situation is not necessarily disastrous, but it does create a limited view of recovery for the client. Naturally therapists are only able to guide their clients through elements of the recovery process that they themselves have resolved in their own personal recovery, or that they feel comfortable with. If, for example, an untreated co-dependent therapist is comfortable working with Emotional Expression, they may exclusively direct the client to do emotional work, always seeking catharsis as the goal of therapy. The result will be an imbalance in the client's recovery. This therapist's client may begin to feel frustrated that they are crying and shouting a lot in therapy but that their behavior and relationships have not appreciably improved.

On the next page is a tool designed to help the recovering couple sustain a consistent and well-balanced recovery together (The Recovery Process Chart). The essence of recovery is the transformation of the Rules of Family Dysfunction into the four healthy Ways of Being. This transformation takes place by applying each of the Elements of Recovery to the dysfunctional rules. In the Recovery Process Chart, the four Rules of Family Dysfunction are listed at the left of the chart. The Elements of Recovery are listed across the top of the chart, and the healthy Ways of Being are listed on the right.

Table 5.1. Recovery Process Chart

Dysfunctional Family Rules	Elements Of Recovery				Healthy Ways Of Being
	Behavioral Action	Emotional Expression	Cognitive Reconstruction	Spiritual Awareness	
Rigidity	Practice letting go of control. Compromise. Change behavior.	Spontaneous release.	I am keeping an open mind.	Whatever God is, my human concept is too small; I am open to learn new ways of experiencing spirituality.	Flexibility

Silence	Talk about what you see, hear and feel.	Face fear, feel repressed feelings.	I am talking about what I feel, see and hear.	I am expressing my spiritual beliefs in the action of my day-to-day life.	**Expression**
Denial	Match inner feeling states with outer expression.	Recognize inner feeling states.	I accept what I see, hear and feel as real.	I accept that there is a spiritual force that works in my life.	**Acceptance**
Isolation	Seek support, make contact with other people.	Honestly express feelings to others.	I am having intimate relationships.	I am sharing my spiritual beliefs and practices with my life partner.	**Intimacy**

In using the Recovery Process Chart as a guide for well-rounded recovery, remember that each of the Elements of Recovery must be applied to each of the Rules of Family Dysfunction (for example, the transformation from Rigidity to Flexibility will include work in *all four* of the Elements of Recovery).

Now we'll look closely at using the Elements of Recovery to facilitate the transformation process. The Recovery Process Chart is used for tracking individual recovery, as well as a couple's recovery. However, the explanations below are directed specifically toward couples working together to create healthier relationships.

Rigidity >> transformed to >> Flexibility

Behavioral Action: *Practice letting go of control. Compromise. Change behavior.* Each partner in the co-dependent relationship must become aware of their particular control issues, and then make the behavioral changes to support their partner's freedom of action and choice. One example of letting go of control would be both partners equally sharing in financial decision-making.

Negotiation and compromise encourage a "win-win" situation rather than a "win-lose" battle between partners. Couples can learn this art from a good couples' counselor, by taking courses in negotiation or by studying about negotiation techniques together. At first couples will want to practice negotiating small decisions, such as picking a movie, before negotiating more emotionally charged issues, such as whether to send their child to a public or a private school.

Act differently. Most rigid behavior patterns are dysfunctional. He can do the housework. She can drive the car when they go out. Whatever your patterns are, try to dismantle these rigid habits and behaviors. Together, look at how you behave as a couple and discuss how to modify some areas of your behavior with each other.

Emotional Expression: *Spontaneous release.* Begin to express your emotions spontaneously with each other. When you are happy, allow yourself to smile and be playful. Practice showing each other what you are feeling while you are feeling it. Notice when you are trying to rigidly control your emotions. If your partner does something to hurt your feelings, try to express the hurt while you are feeling it. Spontaneous release of feelings keeps relationships alive and interesting.

Cognitive Reconstruction: *I am keeping an open mind.* Affirm, both individually and as a couple, that you are open to explore new ways of doing things. When one partner changes behavior, it is most effective when the other partner agrees to be open to that change and does not condemn the new behavior just because it is unfamiliar. When conflict occurs, keeping an open mind is the creative vehicle to a satisfactory solution.

Spiritual Awareness: *Whatever God is, my human concept is too small; I am open to learning new ways of experiencing spirituality.* Many couples bring their past religious prejudices with them into their relationship. As a couple, begin to work at letting go of old inhibiting ideas about spirituality and together explore new approaches. This may mean returning to the religion of your childhood or trying something altogether different. The point is to keep an open mind.

Silence >> transformed to >> Expression

Behavioral Action: *Talk about what you see, hear and feel.* As a couple take time to get together to report how you feel in the relationship. If you see your partner behaving in a way that disturbs you, then say so. This is not the same as blaming or judging. The idea is just to report what you are seeing and how you feel about it. If your partner says one thing, then appears to do another, double-check what your partner means — ask them about it. Continue to report what you see, hear and feel and to check out your interpretations with your partner again and again. This takes practice!

Emotional Expression: *Face fear, feel repressed feelings.* It is unrealistic for either partner to assume they will always be able to report feelings on the spot. At first both partners will feel fear about expressing their emotions. Sometimes the fear will be so great, the emotion will be repressed. Begin to become aware of when this is happening. Facing the fear of expressing your feelings and trusting your partner enough to share the fear, as well as the repressed feelings, is the kind of vulnerability that is necessary for a truly intimate relationship.

Cognitive Reconstruction: *I am talking about what I feel, see and hear.* Affirming that you are being honest with each other about what you are feeling, seeing and hearing in the relationship is a way to encourage each other. It also ensures that it will actually happen. As busy as most of us are, it's easy to let time slip past without really talking to each other. Plan specific times during the week to be together so that this sharing can take place.

Spiritual Awareness: *I am expressing my spiritual beliefs in the actions of my day-to-day life.* When a couple expresses their spirituality together, they plant the seeds for a strong spiritual foundation that will hold the relationship together in times of trouble and challenge. Discussing your spiritual beliefs with your spouse or lover, praying and/or meditating together, attending church or synagogue, "saying grace" before meals and going on spiritual retreats together are a few of the many ways to express your spirituality as a couple.

Denial >>transformed to>>Acceptance

Behavioral Action: *Match inner feeling states with outer expression.* It is easy to mask your inner feeling states. An example of "masking" is smiling when you feel angry or sad or displaying no outward emotional expression at a time when you are feeling strong emotions. You may need support in accepting, rather than denying, your feelings. Your partner can be a great deal of help if you ask them to (gently) point out inconsistencies in what you say you feel and how you appear to be feeling.

Emotional Expression: *Recognize inner feeling states.* Stop and take time to *experience* what you are feeling. Emotional states often pass unrecognized when we have spent years denying or ignoring our feelings. Practice recognizing what you are feeling, and expressing it to your partner. You can help each other to recognize different feelings. At the end of Chapter 3 is a list of feeling statements. You and your partner can use this list as a reference to identify various feeling states.

Cognitive Reconstruction: *I accept what I see, hear and feel as real.* Trust your senses and accept that the information they give you is real. Affirm with your partner that you both accept each other as you are today. Learning to accept the reality of each other's humanness removes unnecessary strain from the relationship.

Spiritual Awareness: *I accept that there is a spiritual force that works in my life.* Accepting a spiritual presence in our lives includes a spiritual presence in our relationships. This guiding force supports our relationships as well as our lives as individuals. Accepting that our life with our partner has purpose and meaning, can be an important bonding experience.

Isolation >> transformed to >> Intimacy

Behavioral Action: *Seek support, make contact with other people.* Develop nurturing friends outside of your primary relationship. Each partner needs strong healthy friendships outside of their relationship with each other. Take action to develop those friendships. Of course, your partner is also your friend, but if your partner is your only friend, you are putting all your eggs in one basket. Sooner or later you will need a good friend to talk to outside the relationship.

Emotional Expression: *Honestly express feelings to others.* When you honestly express feelings to other people, you make emotional contact with them. Without emotional contact, intimacy cannot exist. In friendships, as well as in coupleship, emotional contact is the vehicle that gives a relationship the richness that keeps it stimulating.

Cognitive Reconstruction: *I am having intimate relationships.* Affirm to yourself and with your partner that you are having intimate relationships. Affirm your intimacy in your love relationship and in your friendships. These are relationships you value, that you choose because you want these people to be in your life. Affirm this fact.

Spiritual Awareness: *I am sharing my spiritual beliefs and practices with my life partner.* Spiritual intimacy takes place when you and your partner share spiritual beliefs and practices. When your relationship is founded on spiritual intimacy, your bond with each other will last through difficulties and hardships, and will grow and prosper.

A well-balanced, consistent recovery process is an ideal to work toward. In the reality of daily life, however, recovery is apt to be inconsistent at times. A co-dependent person, learning about emotional expression for the first time, usually begins by focusing most of their energy on being emotionally expressive. There is nothing wrong with this. It is the way most of us learn. At other times we may focus on behavioral action. The goal is to integrate each of the Elements of Recovery into the process so that recovery touches every area of our lives. The time and manner in which this integration takes place is somewhat different for each of us.

The recovering couple can use the Recovery Process Chart to assist them in bringing healthy growth to their interactions with each other. Usually partners will work on different personal issues at different times. Differences need not cause despair or discontent in the relationship. In fact, they often strengthen the relationship. When we know our partner is working on recovery just as we are, we have an opportunity to extend to them the kind of loving support that occurs in every healthy relationship. These active expressions of intimacy help us heal together.

Following is a blank copy of the Recovery Process Chart. Make copies of this chart, and fill it in with your own needs and goals. Be creative in your application of the chart. There is no right or wrong way to use it. Let it be a guide to recovery and transformation.

Table 5.2. Recovery Process Chart

Dysfunctional Family Rules	Elements Of Recovery				Healthy Ways Of Being
	Behavioral Action	Emotional Expression	Cognitive Reconstruction	Spiritual Awareness	
Rigidity					Flexibility

Expression	Acceptance	Intimacy
Silence	Denial	Isolation

6

Types Of Co-dependent Relationships

Co-dependent relationships are problematic because like the dysfunctional family system, they are based on fear. Co-dependent people in such relationships can be described in two categories: those who primarily experience the *fear of abandonment* with their partners, and those who primarily experience the *fear of engulfment*. These two ways of relating have their roots in the co-dependent's childhood experiences of dysfunctional living. Knowing how these two fears, abandonment and engulfment, adversely affect sexual relationships, can help co-dependents understand better their sometimes puzzling feelings and behaviors.

The following diagram is designed to help you understand these two important fear states and their effects in co-dependent sexual relationships.

**Figure 6.1. The Origin Of Abandonment And Engulfment
In Co-dependent Relationships**

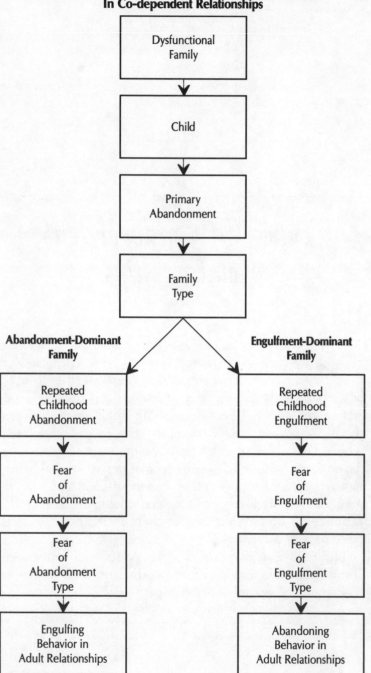

Dysfunctional Family

The dysfunctional family cannot supply healthy support and love to its members. It operates according to the four dysfunctional rules we discussed earlier: Denial, Silence, Isolation and Rigidity. At the core of the dysfunctional family is any one of a variety of compulsive/addictive diseases or disorders such as alcoholism, eating disorders or sexual abuse.

Child

A child becomes part of a dysfunctional family by being born into it, being adopted into it or having a parent who marries into it. The child is not the cause of dysfunction in the family. The child is powerless over the dysfunction and the actions of the adults in the family. It is the responsibility of adults to protect, nurture and provide safety for children. Children are not safe in dysfunctional families. The more dysfunctional the family, the more hazardous it is for the child.

Primary Abandonment

Primary abandonment occurs during the first three years of childhood and is experienced by the adult co-dependent as a feeling of emptiness, a "hole in the soul" or intense fear of loneliness. Primary abandonment is a core experience for all co-dependents, stemming from a parent or parents' emotional unavailability. When a baby is born into a dysfunctional family, the family's focus is on the source of dysfunction not on the child. An infant born into this system does not get the consistent nurturing and attention necessary to feel safe and secure. A child will experience this lack of nurturing as terrifying abandonment.

Although primary abandonment always involves emotional distance and neglect, it sometimes includes physical abandonment and neglect. Some examples of physical abandonment are missed feedings, unchanged diapers and being left alone for long periods of time. Emotional and physical abandonment seriously damage a child's development, leaving them with a core of fear. Later as this person enters adult relationships, the fear of being abandoned remains, even though they may not consciously recognize it. All people from dysfunctional families have primary abandonment issues.

Family Type

A dysfunctional family will either abandon or engulf its children. The pattern established by the family (whether abandoning or engulfing) has a profound effect on the children's adult sexual relationships. This pattern leads to the development of either the Abandonment-Dominant Family or the Engulfment-Dominant Family.

Abandonment-Dominant Family

In this family parents are so absorbed in the central dysfunction (alcoholism, eating disorders, etc.) that the children are ignored. These parents have neither emotional energy nor time (two crucial developmental needs) to devote to their children. They are so preoccupied with trying to control the dysfunction, they are unable to meet the emotional, and sometimes the physical, needs of their children. The abandonment-dominant family establishes a consistent pattern of emotional distance between parent and child. Children are often treated as objects that are inconvenient and in the way. Co-dependents raised in such a family received this message: "You are in the way and we would be better off without you."

Repeated Childhood Abandonment

Abandonment becomes a way of life for the children in this family system. Because they are not able to establish real emotional contact with their parents, their parent-child bond is at best faulty. A childhood spent in this family is a series of disappointments and broken promises. Parents do not actively participate in their children's lives, except as they relate to what the parents themselves are doing at any given moment. The children are left to their own resources. Throughout their childhood, their parents forget to pick them up at school, do not show up at recitals and school plays and break promise after promise. The parents often agree to do things for their children out of guilt, then neglect to follow through.

In many cases abandonment accompanies a shocking level of carelessness. When Bill was a child, he came home from school one afternoon to a house that was completely bare of furniture. His parents had moved during the day. At the age of 11, Bill went to a neighbor, got his new address and traveled by himself to where his parents had moved — *six miles across town*. His parents had moved his belongings, and his things were set up in his room, but no one had thought to tell him of the impending move. Until Bill entered therapy, he had never mentioned to anyone this unnerving experience of being abandoned by his parents.

Fear Of Abandonment

Children never get used to being abandoned. No matter how often abandonment happens, it hurts, and children never lose hope that maybe this time it will be different. As a child matures through adolescence and teenage years, repeated parental abandonment takes its toll. The child begins to feel that no place is safe in the world, and that he or she must be in control to feel safe. The child knows what it is to be forgotten. The child who is repeatedly abandoned knows the sinking feeling when a parent is emotionally absent. Children feel their emotions very intensely and deeply. When they are abandoned, either physically or emotionally, their hurt and pain stays with them.

Fear Of Abandonment Type

A co-dependent who has fear of abandonment at the center of their adult relationships shows the characteristics of the Fear of Abandonment Type. This person's fear is often so powerful that they believe, at some level, that they might die if the relationship ended. The Fear of Abandonment Type will tolerate almost anything to keep their relationship together: physical and emotional abuse and loss of self-respect and self-worth. They are driven by their fear of loneliness and their need to have someone in their life whom they believe might be able to fill the void they feel inside themselves.

Engulfing Behavior In Adult Relationships

The fear of abandonment and the need to feel secure leads co-dependents to engulfing behavior in relationships. Fear of Abandonment Types *engulf*, or smother, their partner in an attempt to prevent re-experiencing their childhood feelings of abandonment. A relationship that centers around a fear of its dissolution is never healthy. Constant fear is unhealthy. The Fear of Abandonment Type believes that controlling their partner will alleviate their pain. In the words of one co-dependent, "I thought that if I could completely control my husband, I would be safe because then he would never be able to leave me. I would be in control."

But ironically the fear that compels the co-dependent to this engulfing behavior is itself very painful. Perpetual worry about controlling our partner is not any more comfortable than feeling abandoned. Some examples of engulfing behaviors are: an obsessive need to know the whereabouts of our partner, attempting to control and manipulate our partner's behavior, appearing helpless, clinging to our partner and trying to become indispensable.

Engulfment-Dominant Family

As a distraction from the pain and fear of its central dysfunctions (alcoholism, eating disorders, etc.), the parents in this system focus all of their attention on their child. The parents in the Engulfment-Dominant Family overwhelm their child with their emotional and sometimes physical, needs. The parents habitually use their child to diffuse their own pain and to boost their own wounded sense of self-worth. In this system the child's boundaries are repeatedly violated. They are treated as non-persons who are an extension of their parents. The message these children receive is: "You exist only to meet our needs, and you will do what we want you to do. Your needs and desires are unimportant."

Repeated Childhood Engulfment

Engulfment is a way of life for a child raised in this family. Their parents constantly violate their sense of self. Because of the overwhelming emotional pressure placed upon this child, developing a personal identity is difficult. The parents exert their control over every aspect of the child's life, telling them how to dress, whom they may have as friends, what to feel. These children are often forced, or intimidated into, participating in activities they do not want to be involved in. The child may say, "I like the color blue," and the mother will respond, "No you don't. You've always liked red better than blue."

"My parents said I had a choice about what I wanted to take in school. But I really didn't," said Allen, a recovering co-dependent. "If I didn't take the courses they suggested, they wouldn't talk to me, or they would start to nag me about little things that really didn't matter. I learned a long time ago just to do what my parents wanted me to, or they would make my life miserable. Not just in school but in every part of my life. I've never really felt I had a life of my own."

Fear Of Engulfment

Children who are engulfed by their parents are threatened with loss of self. When children do not learn to make decisions, or to test their emerging egos, their sense of who they are as human beings is smothered. It is the job of parents to assist their children in discovering their own unique characteristics and strengths and to teach them how to make their own healthy decisions (not to make their decisions for them). Instead engulfing parents repress their child's sense of self. The child is taught to respond to the parent's needs, while ignoring their own needs. Children know intuitively that their parents are wrong to smother them. They know and feel that the engulfment threatens their freedom to be individual human beings, separate from their parents. Children who are engulfed are robbed of their birthright to be themselves. It is no wonder that when these children reach adulthood, they have a deep fear of being swallowed up by their spouse or lover. Many such people interpret requests for intimacy as a threat to their identity.

Fear Of Engulfment Type

A Fear of Engulfment Type primarily fears being engulfed or consumed by their partner. This fear is often strong enough to drive them from one relationship to another in a long series of hasty escapes. Each time they end a relationship, this person feels as if they got out just in time. The Fear of Engulfment Type feels extremely threatened by others' attempts at closeness and intimacy. Their fear keeps them emotionally distant and suspicious of their partner. They need and want intimacy as much as anyone else does, but intimacy is also their primary fear.

Abandoning Behavior In Adult Relationships

The fear of engulfment, and the perceived need to protect one's sense of self, results in abandoning behavior in relationships. The Fear of Engulfment Type abandons their partner when the relationship begins to trigger the feelings of engulfment they felt with their parents. This person's fear of engulfment is intense. They feel as if their selfhood, their uniqueness, will be absorbed by their partner, and they will disappear. In order to protect against this loss of self, the Fear of Engulfment Type continually places distance, both emotional and physical, between themselves and their partner.

Physical distancing can include an unwillingness to touch or hug, becoming emotionally or sexually unavailable or leaving the relationship altogether. Emotional unavailability, or emotional abandonment, involves not honestly expressing feelings or using emotional excesses (such as explosive rage) to frighten one's partner. To scare off a partner, the Fear of Engulfment Type may throw things or sob hysterically. Whatever the pattern, all the abandoning behaviors have their basis in an intense fear that one's individuality will be wiped out completely.

Three Types Of Co-dependent Relationships

The two primary fears of the co-dependent, abandonment and engulfment, create three basic types of co-dependent relationships. These are:

1. **The Abandonment/Engulfment Relationship**
2. **The Abandonment/Abandonment Relationship**
3. **The Engulfment/Engulfment Relationship**

This is a set of models to help us consider patterns that generally occur in co-dependent relationships. Few relationships will purely and completely fit any one of these models.

The Abandonment/Engulfment Relationship

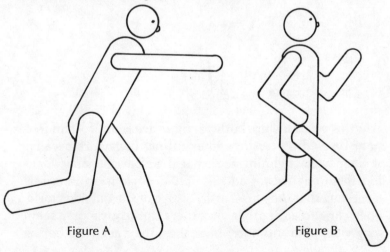

Figure A   Figure B

This relationship joins a Fear of Abandonment (FOA) Type with a Fear of Engulfment (FOE) Type. The FOA Type engulfs their partner in an attempt to prevent feeling abandoned (figure A). The FOE Type, overwhelmed by their partner's engulfing behavior, acts out their fear by abandoning them (figure B). This abandonment creates more fear in the FOA partner, who responds with even more intense engulfing behavior.

Each partner is acting out of their primary fear and is unable to get their desire for intimacy fulfilled. One partner (FOA) is always involved in chasing the other (FOE) partner, who is always escaping. This relationship is frustrating for both people.

The Engulfment/Engulfment Relationship

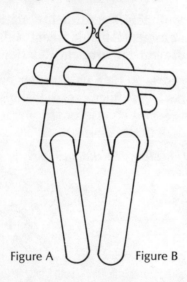

Figure A   Figure B

In this relationship, both partners are Fear of Abandonment types. Both engage in engulfing behaviors because of their overwhelming fear that their partner may abandon them (figures A and B). This couple is so intensely enmeshed that they are hardly aware of the outside world. They cling to each other. To others, this couple may seem very close and intimate; in reality, they are smothering each other. This relationship has a desperate quality. It is unable to grow or to change. Changes in behavior are perceived by either partner as an indication that the other is about to leave. The partners stay locked in the relationship, both paralyzed by their fear.

The Abandonment/Abandonment Relationship

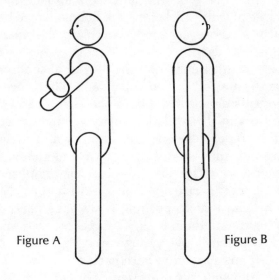

Figure A   Figure B

Both partners in this relationship are afraid of disappearing into their partner. They act out their fear of engulfment by abandoning (figures A and B). This couple keep each other at arm's length. Neither is willing to risk being vulnerable. They often appear to have little in common and live fairly separate lives. Outside observers frequently marvel that this couple, so distant from each other, stay together. The fact that they stay together indicates their genuine desire to be intimate, though their fear of engulfment continues to prevent them from bonding intimately with each other. There is no intimacy and no emotional contact in this relationship. The couple are only comfortable when each partner remains at a safe distance.

Summary

In the search for a happy and fulfilling relationship, the co-dependent may move from one type of relationship to another. It is not unusual for someone to move out of an Abandonment/Engulfment relationship into an Abandonment/Abandonment Relationship and then back again. Escaping from one type of relationship into another does not produce a healthy relationship. Relationships based in fear, such as those depicted above, are destined to be unfulfilling and dysfunctional.

Primary abandonment and the fear of abandonment is always an issue for the co-dependent. Therefore, some co-dependents demonstrate both abandoning and engulfing behaviors in their relationships. A person raised in a family that repeatedly engulfed them will also have to work through the issue of primary abandonment. Many times people who act on their fear of engulfment by abandoning their partner, will also feel a fear of abandonment. This can lead to pushing away one's partner, and then trying to pull them back. This message is sometimes referred to as the "I love you, go away" phenomenon and is confusing and painful to both partners.

The relationship types presented in this chapter are based upon what I have observed in clinical practice with adult co-dependents. However, human experience is varied and complex. While these categories can help us understand general trends in co-dependent relationships, it is certain that some couples will not match the model exactly (thank heaven). Our unique qualities are what make us human beings so interesting and delightful. If you can use this information, and if it eases your understanding of problems or difficulties you may be having in relationships, then it has served its purpose. If you feel that none of these models applies to you, trust your intuition.

The root of dysfunction in all three types of co-dependent relationships is fear. When the fear is resolved and replaced with love and with healthy new behavior, these relationships can become joyful and richly satisfying.

7

Bonding In The Sexual Relationship

Within each human being is a desire to become profoundly intimate with another person. This desire to be in a deep union, or *bonded*, in a love relationship is a healthy and natural aspect of human existence. It is an experience that can both enrich and reward the lives of both partners in ways that cannot be imagined, only experienced.

In a bonded relationship there is a deep sense of connection with another human being in a way that transcends other kinds of relationships. The risks in this relationship are also great: frustration, confusion and pain can also be felt very deeply. But even though it involves taking risks, many people feel the lack of an intimate love relationship as a loneliness and isolation that cannot be erased.

Co-dependents are no different from other people in their desire for a special intimate relationship. The co-dependent, however, brings to their relationship a set of problems unique to growing up in a dysfunctional environment. Having taken a close look at the dysfunctional family system, it is easy to see why sexual relationships are difficult for co-dependents. But while having a healthy relationship may be challenging for co-dependent people, it is not impossible. The key word is "healthy." Many co-dependents are involved in sexual relationships. Unfortunately their relationships are often shallow and unfulfilling. Co-dependent relationships seem to be an ongoing cycle of pain or end in a painful mess. When their relationships end, they often find themselves almost immediately in another relationship that eventually ends in the same way. This frustrating pattern does not have to continue. The cycle can be broken by a willingness to learn and to change.

It is important that co-dependents understand that a lack of knowledge about healthy relationships is not a hopeless character flaw. If co-dependents learned the dysfunctional family rules, they can also unlearn them. There is, of course, quite a lot to learn.

Some examples of the skills necessary to healthy relationships are:

How to communicate honestly about how they feel,

How to tell the difference between bonding and "blending" with another person, and

How to know the difference between solitude and isolation.

The many areas where change is needed can be overwhelming. It is important to keep in mind that we cannot learn everything at once; learning takes time and repetition. Even for healthy people, learning the dance of relationship is a lifetime process. But it is encouraging to see how quickly a relationship will begin to heal once both partners make a firm commitment to health and begin to experiment by relating to each other in new ways.

Basic to moving toward a healthier relationship is the understanding that *both partners are equal.* One person in the relationship is not sicker or healthier than the other. Each person may have difficulties in relationships, but neither of them deserves blame. Both partners must share responsibility for the difficulties and successes they have as a couple.

Being involved in a healthy growth-centered sexual relationship is an exciting experience. Essential to this experience is our ability to bond with our partner.

Bonding is deep, intimate contact with another person. This intense contact includes physical expression (touching, sex), emotional connections shared at a deep level of trust and openness, and mental connections that include sharing ideas and beliefs with our partner. When people bond with each other, they are making a commitment to share themselves at a deep level and to acknowledge that their relationship is an integrated part of their spiritual life.

Co-dependents often have a tendency to confuse bonding with blending. Bonding is the process of deepening the relationship between two people, in which both the relationship and the individuals in the relationship become stronger and more balanced. When *blending* occurs, however, each person gets lost in the relationship by attempting in various ways to control the other person (to re-establish their own lost sense of security and individuality). Bonding strengthens both the couple and the individuals; blending cripples both the couple and the individuals.

An Exercise In Bonding

This is a bonding exercise for couples who are already in
a committed sexual relationship and who wish to deepen
that relationship by connecting with their partner at deeper
levels of experience. This exercise is most effective when
it is practiced regularly over a period of time. Please read
through the instructions together before you begin.

First, make sure that you will not be disturbed for
the next hour. Take the phone off the hook, put out the
"Do Not Disturb" sign, make sure the kids are asleep
or gone, put out the cat. Make the room as safe and
soft as possible. Turn down the lights, perhaps light a
candle or two. Play some soft meditative music (without
lyrics). The exercise produces best results when both
partners are nude (so be sure the room is warm
enough). However, since opening and deepening often
includes feelings of vulnerability, wearing clothing may
feel more comfortable the first few times you and your
partner try this bonding exercise together.

Begin with you and your partner sitting, either on
chairs or on the floor, closely facing each other, but
without touching. Say nothing. Just relax and be still.

As you sit looking at each other, become aware of
your breathing as it flows in and out of your body. As
you become aware of your own natural breathing cycle,
notice also your partner's breathing cycle. Gradually
begin to synchronize the breathing between the two of
you. Let your breath move in harmony, both of you
breathing in and out as one.

Hold eye contact with each other for two or three
minutes. Remember that this is a bonding experience,
not a stare-down. It is all right to blink (eyes need to
blink, blinking is healthy). Continue to breathe together.

As you look into each other's eyes, become aware of
your partner's face. Let your eyes roam freely around
your partner's face. Lovingly study your partner's face.
Become aware of all face parts: the nose, the area

around the eyes, the eyelids, the forehead, the mouth, cheeks and hair. Look at the details of your partner's face, the crinkles at the corner of the eyes and mouth, the pores of the skin. Be aware, and love, any feature that makes the face unique, such as birthmarks, dimples, perhaps a scar. Really study, really see, the face of the one you love. Do this for approximately 10 minutes. Remember to continue breathing together.

At this point, either partner may slowly and gently place the palm of their right hand on the heart of their partner. Then the other person mirrors this action by placing the palm of their right hand on the heart of their partner. Now that you are both touching your partner's heart area, place your left hand on your own heart area, over your partner's hand.

The two of you are now sitting facing each other, looking at each other, touching, and breathing together as one. *(It is often helpful to practice the positioning of the hands before you try this bonding experience for the first time.)*

Now sit in this position for approximately 15 minutes (it is all right to use a clock). As you are sitting like this, communicate your love to your partner with your eyes and through your hands.

At the end of approximately 15 minutes, gently disengage your hands. End the experience by saying the affirmation, "I love myself, and I love you."

Remain still for a few minutes together before sharing what each of you experienced during this bonding exercise.

This is often a very powerful experience for both partners. Sometimes the feelings that arise during this experience can even be painful and frightening. True bonding with another can be scary. Do not become discouraged if painful feelings of hurt, anger, fear, shame and guilt arise during this experience. Make an agreement with your partner, before you begin this exercise, that either one of you may end the exercise early if you wish.

If the exercise ends early, don't worry about it. You did not do it wrong. Agree to try it again later.

The above experience can produce remarkable results in deepening a relationship. Bonding is important. Without a healthy bond, the couple in the relationship will not experience the deep sense of contact and connectedness that set the sexual relationship apart from other relationships. Still, the exercise is only an experience. What makes it work is the love and willingness of the couple to explore new realms of being and sharing.

Co-dependents have love and willingness in abundance. What they lack is knowledge about how to share the love and willingness that they already possess. Bonding, as well as the other skills necessary to a healthy relationship, can be learned. The challenge to the co-dependent is twofold. First, we must learn the skills essential to a healthy, loving relationship. Second, we must acknowledge the gifts we already possess, and allow those gifts to begin to unfold in loving and healthy ways.

8

Survivors Of Sexual Abuse And Their Partners

Sexual drive and the desire for physical intimacy is a powerful force in the recovering relationship. The sexual attraction between partners can be a wonderful bonding experience. Although sexual desire is a natural and healthy aspect of adult relationships, it is important to be aware that our sexual behavior, emotional responses to sex and attitudes about sex are significantly shaped by our past sexual experiences. Having been sexually abused directly affects our sexuality.

Because each person in a recovering co-dependent relationship comes from a dysfunctional family, there is a strong likelihood that one, or even both, have experienced childhood sexual abuse. Alcoholic families, for example, have a much higher incidence of childhood sexual abuse than other families. If either member of the relationship has a history of sexual abuse, it will have a profound effect on the relationship.

For co-dependent people (and often for others as well), a curtain of secrecy, silence and repression surrounds the subject of childhood sexual abuse. It is not easily talked about. The co-dependent who was sexually abused as a child often has either repressed the memory, or claims the abuse had no effect on them. In either case unresolved sexual abuse issues have a serious impact on both the individual and the relationship. Until childhood sexual abuse is treated, it is as though the survivor of that abuse were living on top of a volcano, with the ever-present potential for a devastating explosion of repressed emotions.

Ironically co-dependents involved in recovering relationships frequently find that their growing intimacy and trust encourages these painful sexual abuse issues to rise to the surface. Safe at last, the survivor finds that their painful memories of childhood sexual abuse return to be dealt with. The walls of repression begin to break down in the loving atmosphere of recovery. As trust evolves in the recovering relationship, the sexual abuse survivor feels safe enough to remember what happened and to feel their deeply repressed feelings. This marks the entry into an even deeper level of recovery, both for the survivor and their partner.

Strong emotional responses to the issues of sexual abuse can create havoc in a relationship. During the process of recovery from sexual trauma, sexual activity between the couple will almost certainly change and extreme emotional experiences are normal. The abuse survivor re-experiences intense feelings of betrayal and abandonment that they had stored inside since childhood, as well as powerful feelings of shame, fear, hurt and rage. Unfortunately these intense feelings are sometimes directed toward their partner, especially if the survivor strongly trusts their partner.

In the initial stages of recovery from sexual abuse, the couple may feel that their relationship is doomed. A feeling of distrust and emotional distance may temporarily come between them. The recovering couple can survive this challenge, however, and turn the experience into an opportunity to build trust and intimacy in the relationship. There is no avoiding the fact that dealing with sexual abuse issues, as well as supporting one's partner in recovery from such damaging experiences, is very difficult work. These issues test the strength of the healthiest relationship, and faith is required for partners to maintain their intimacy in the face of such a challenge. Not only will the survivor of sexual abuse need to work on their sexual issues, but their partner (also raised in dysfunction) will become aware of unhealthy sexual attitudes and behaviors they also may have, as well as other areas where recovery is still needed.

During the intense period of recovery from sexual trauma, it is essential that each of the partners *seek support outside of the relationship*. Each partner must have a place to vent their feelings and express their thoughts without having to censor what they say. Whether they go to friends, therapists, clergy or other people they trust, it is absolutely necessary that both partners seek outside support if the relationship is to remain strong.

The sexual abuse survivors must also find for themselves a safe place where their feelings and memories will be validated by others. Dealing with childhood sexual abuse is extremely painful. No one should have to face it alone. A professional therapist trained in the treatment of sexual trauma is of great assistance in guiding survivors through the special challenges of their recovery.

Types Of Childhood Sexual Abuse

There is usually so much denial, secrecy and memory loss surrounding childhood sexual abuse that it is important to discuss, at least briefly, types of sexual abuse. The following is not intended to be a comprehensive work on sexual trauma, but an informative overview to help recovering couples recognize childhood sexual abuse in their history. (If this information does not answer your questions, please refer to the Bibliography for suggestions for further reading.)

The most commonly recognized situation of childhood sexual abuse is a father abusing his female child. Sexual abuse, however, is not limited to this particular model, and certainly not just to incest situations. Fathers also sexually abuse their male children, and mothers sexually abuse their male and female children. Physically stronger brothers and sisters can sexually abuse their weaker and younger siblings. In families where such abuse exists, a child is often abused by more than one family member.

One man I worked with was forced by his older brother to have sex with his eight-year-old sister. Both his older brother and his father had regularly abused his sister, and they wanted to involve him in the sexual abuse. Children in dysfunctional families are often poorly protected by their parents, and are easy targets for abusers who are not members of the immediate family.

There are two kinds of sexual abuse: *overt* abuse and *covert* abuse. Each has devastating effects on children.

Overt Sexual Abuse

Overt sexual abuse takes place when an adult physically uses a child for sexual gratification. This includes forcing a child to perform oral sex and having anal or vaginal sex with a child. Anal, oral and vaginal sex with children are the most commonly recognized forms of overt sexual abuse. Other kinds of overt sexual abuse include fondling or penetrating the child's anus or vagina with fingers or objects such as sexual aids, broom handles, hair brushes or other objects. Inappropriate (sexual) bathing, hugging and kissing of children also fall under the category of overt abuse. Certain invasive "medical" or "health" procedures may also be overt sexual abuse.

Tom's mother, an alcoholic, gave him and his sister two enemas every day until he was nine years old. He reported that his sister, two years younger than he, was also vaginally douched each day. This sexual abuse began when Tom and his sister were very young. Tom's mother stopped abusing him when he was old enough to physically stop her. He entered therapy because he would sometimes experience feelings of rage toward his wife during sexual foreplay. He was also having such intense feelings of rage toward his mother that he thought he might physically harm her.

Although Tom was not aware of his mother having any sexual gratification when she was abusing him and his sister, nevertheless, what his mother did to him and to his sister was overt sexual abuse. Over a period of time, Tom's rage at his mother decreased in intensity and he learned not to direct these old feelings toward his wife.

Other kinds of overt sexual abuse of a child have to do with non-physical contact with an adult. This abuse includes the adult sexually exposing him or herself, masturbating in front of the child, having sex with another adult in front of the child and forcing or encouraging the child to masturbate in front of the adult. There are many other types of overt sexual abuse, such as taking sexually suggestive pictures of children and forcing or encouraging a child to have sex with other children.

Sexual abuse can cause physical trauma, as well as emotional trauma, for survivors. An adult man who penetrates a child's vagina or anus with his penis can cause a great deal of physical pain and trauma to the child.

One man I worked with was forced to have oral sex with his older step-brother. Sometimes during this forced sex, he would choke and gag so violently that he would lose consciousness.

Covert Sexual Abuse

Covert sexual abuse, sometimes called "emotional incest," occurs when there is sexually-charged emotional interaction, usually between a parent and a child. Covert sexual abuse often does not involve physical sexual contact, but its effects are seriously damaging to the child. Basic to covert sexual abuse is the phenomenon of parent/child sexual equalization. The parent acts as if the child is a sexual equal (treats the child as an adult), and uses the child to meet their *emotional* need for a sexual partner. A common example occurs when parents use their child as a confidante, disclosing information about their sexual frustrations and their sexual activity. Such behavior is inappropriate in the parent/child relationship and forces the child to take on an adult sexual role with the parent.

When a mother elevates her son to the position of "man of the house" and talks to him about her sexual problems with her husband or her lover, she is covertly sexually abusing him. Her son is placed in the damaging position of providing emotional support and sexual understanding beyond his years, as well as assuming the inappropriate role of caretaker to his mother, rather than being cared for by her. This confusing behavior on the part of a parent causes a child to reach adulthood with deep feelings of sexual inadequacy and insecurity. The same is true for the female child who becomes her father's little girlfriend. Even if her father does not speak to her about his sex life or sexual feelings but treats his daughter like a surrogate spouse (taking her out on dates as he would an adult woman or expecting her to fulfill a wifely role), he is covertly sexually abusing her. Any time a parent uses their child to get their emotional sexual needs met, covert sexual abuse is occurring. The healthy adult will seek out another adult to confide in, rather than abuse their child in this way.

Covert sexual abuse in childhood seriously affects the adult co-dependent's sexual relationships. The survivor feels emotionally and sexually unequal to their partner. This feeling of futility springs from their childhood attempts to provide an adult kind of emotional support for their parents at a time when it was beyond their capabilities.

One woman in therapy summed up her feelings about being covertly abused: "I hated it when my father told me about his sexual frustration with my mother. I just wanted to be his little girl; I didn't want to know all that stuff. It made me feel like I should do something for my father, but I didn't know what. I felt inadequate and confused then, and now I feel the same way with my husband. At least now I know where these feelings came from and I can work on letting them go."

Another form of covert sexual abuse that frequently occurs in dysfunctional families is sexual shaming. Children who are ridiculed regarding a natural curiosity about their bodies often develop deep feelings of embarrassment and shame. As adults these people frequently have difficulty talking to their partners about sex and are embarrassed about the physical appearance of their bodies.

Although sexual shaming can begin at any age for the child, it sometimes becomes more intense during puberty. Parents who are insecure about their own sexuality, and are ashamed of their own bodies, often ridicule, tease and shame their children during puberty. While respectful humor and laughter is healthy in a family, the dysfunctional family's jokes and teasing are often degrading and damage the maturing child's sexual self-image. Some parents use dirty jokes and inappropriate sexual teasing to deal with their own fear and insecurity about their child's emerging sexuality.

One day in therapy Stacy told her group that her father had teased her about her body when she had started to mature physically. He teased and joked about her breast size and made fun of her when she had her period. When Stacy began to date, the shaming got worse. Every time she brought a boyfriend home, her father would make fun of her in this degrading way. She became so embarrassed that she refused to bring boys home. To exert control Stacy's father then made a rule that she could not date anyone whom he had not met. This effectively stopped her from dating. She told the group, "I began to sneak out of the house at night to meet boys. Since I believed I was a bad girl anyway, I had sex with anyone who asked. Even today I feel like sex is sort of dirty and bad and I get very embarrassed when anyone tells a joke that is even remotely sexual."

Covert sexual abuse also occurs in the area of punishment. Children are sometimes punished by being forced to take their clothes off when their parents spank them or beat them. Aside from the fact that hitting is almost always physically abusive, shaming a child by exposing their nakedness makes this physical abuse sexual in nature. If a child is punished in this manner while other people (adults or children) are present, their embarrassment and shame is compounded.

At a certain point in their development, children will express a desire for privacy while bathing, dressing, going to the toilet and doing other personal activities. When a parent continually violates the child's boundaries by walking in unannounced at these times, covert sexual abuse is occurring.

There are many subtle ways in which children are covertly sexually abused. Many parents (themselves children of dysfunction) covertly sexually abuse their children without knowing what they are doing. These parents treat their own children as they were treated by their own parents. Parents with unresolved childhood sexual trauma have damaged personal boundaries and may unconsciously sexually abuse their children. Although abuse may be unintentional, ignorance on the part of the perpetrator does not lessen the damage to the child, nor to the adult that child will someday become.

If You Are A Sexual Abuse Survivor . . .

Find a support group that you can talk to about the specifics of your sexual abuse. This support group must include other survivors of childhood sexual abuse. Other survivors will be able to understand you and support your recovery. They will be able to validate your feelings and memories. It is not enough to say you have been sexually abused and are hurt and angry about it (even though this is difficult enough by itself). For recovery to take place, you must speak explicitly about the details of your experience with a person or persons who can guide you through your feelings about it.

I strongly recommend working on your sexual abuse issues with a skilled and knowledgeable therapist. It is important to interview the therapist to get a feeling for (1) whether you feel comfortable with them personally, and (2) whether they know what they are doing. Talking to former clients of a therapist can be very helpful to you in selecting your own therapist.

In the beginning of recovery from childhood sexual abuse, it is often best not to tell your partner detailed accounts of your sexual trauma. You may not get the support from him or her that you need and deserve. This does not mean that your partner does not care; they just may not be ready to handle emotionally the details of the abuse. You are not protecting your partner by excluding details from them; *you are protecting yourself*. There may be a time in your recovery when you will want to tell your partner the details but take your time. There is no need to rush.

A sexual abuse survivor named Anne reported that her husband was very supportive when she began to regain the memory that she had been sexually abused. However, when she told him in detail about an incident where her father tied her up and raped her, he could not emotionally handle it. He had to leave the room. Anne said, "I wound up trying to take care of his feelings, rather than getting the validation and support I wanted. Now I tell him the general direction of my treatment and leave the details out. It works a lot better."

Sometimes your partner may want to know the details of your abuse. Only tell your partner if you want to tell them. If your partner pushes you to be explicit, make it clear that you don't want to talk about your abuse. It can be an intimate and rewarding experience to share your experiences in detail with your partner, but it is important to choose a point in your recovery when both of you are ready to do this.

If Your Partner Is A Sexual Abuse Survivor . . .

Your partner is going through a very intense period of recovery. He or she is remembering and re-experiencing a very painful time in their life. It is important to be supportive of your partner, to be emotionally available for them. It is also important to take care of yourself during this time. It is easy to get caught in the emotional whirlwind of sexual abuse recovery and forget about your own needs. Take time for yourself, talk to friends. You may decide to seek professional counseling. Watching a loved one go through so much pain will often cause you to have unhealthy reactions (like either abandoning or engulfing your partner) that are linked to your own dysfunctional childhood. With that in mind, this time can be fertile ground for you to discover and work through some of your own issues.

Your sexual activity with your partner is almost sure to change. It is not uncommon for sexual activity to stop for a period of time. While your partner is re-experiencing their sexual trauma, their sexual desire may disappear. It is important to realize that this is a temporary condition. It probably will not last. Childhood sexual abuse survivors were sexually used and hurt as children. Your partner's sexual trust was broken during childhood and the re-emergence of sex in your relationship can be a part of integrating their healing experience. When you and your partner begin to have sex again, it will be an act of trust, love and faith.

The kind of sexual activity you have had in your relationship may also change. Tony reported in group that he and his wife, Diane, had engaged in oral sex as a regular part of their sex life. During therapy, she remembered her father abusing her by performing oral sex on her and then forcing her to perform oral sex on him. Quite understandably, Diane lost all desire for oral sex while she was processing this information and became furious at Tony when he even suggested oral sex to her. Although the issue of oral sex resolved itself after a time, both partners had some hurt feelings about it. There is nothing wrong with having specific sexual desires. It is, however, abusive to try to manipulate your partner into sexual behaviors they do not wish to engage in. If frustrations arise due to a difference in the frequency or nature of your sexual relations with your partner, talk about your feelings with someone you trust outside the relationship.

During recovery from sexual abuse, your partner will need to learn to set sexual boundaries. In childhood your partner's boundaries were violated, and it is important for your partner to learn that they have control over their own bodies. While your partner is learning to set physical boundaries and limits, he or she may want to change the way you relate to each other sexually. This is your opportunity to watch for feelings of loss of control over your sex life. What is happening is that your partner is trusting you by being completely honest about what they want and don't want sexually. Your partner's willingness to risk in this area can help bring you both into sexual equality with each other, giving both of you a richer and fuller sex life together.

During this time it is natural for you to become extremely angry at the person or persons who sexually abused your partner. It is also common to get angry and resentful at your partner for having sexual abuse in their history. They may not be rational but your emotions are real. Dealing with them is your responsibility and an important ongoing part of your own recovery.

If Both Of You Are Sexual Abuse Survivors . . .

You will both need the strong support of friends and probably therapists. Beware of focusing on your partner's issues rather than on your own. It's easy for co-dependents to do this. Be gentle and tolerant with yourself as well as with your partner. Inevitably there will be times when both of you will need support and understanding at the same time. At these times especially, you will need to go outside the relationship for encouragement and a listening ear. Recovery from childhood sexual abuse is a difficult challenge. Your partner can become an ally and friend who will be able to relate to, and validate, your own experience of sexual abuse. A deep bond can form between you and your partner as a result of having shared a common history of sexual abuse and of sharing in the recovery process. I would suggest re-reading the sections of this chapter entitled, "If Your Partner Is A Sexual Abuse Survivor . . ." and "If You Are A Sexual Abuse Survivor . . ." Since you are both a survivor and the partner of a survivor, you need to know how to respond to both situations.

Summary

Childhood sexual abuse, whether overt or covert, always has an impact on our adult lives, particularly in the area of sexual relationships. Being raised in a dysfunctional family system increases the likelihood of being sexually abused. The more dysfunctional the family, the greater the likelihood. Dealing with childhood sexual abuse is a very intense experience for both partners, and it is likely that the relationship will undergo some difficult changes.

Having a history of childhood sexual abuse does not need to cripple a relationship. The recovering couple can turn the healing of sexual trauma into a deep bonding experience in which both partners increase their love and trust for each other. But the process takes time and work. Sexual abuse issues do not disappear in a week or even in a few months. Begin to develop a realistic view of recovery as a lifelong process. This does not mean that your relationship will be disrupted forever. Healing does occur but in its own time. The support and understanding of a loving partner, and the power of a committed relationship, can greatly facilitate the healing process.

An Exercise

A nonthreatening nonsexual loving way for you and your partner to touch and nurture each other is to give and receive a foot massage. The foot massage gives physical touch and caring without sexual expectations. The feet are generally "sexually safe" for physical touch, and are also an intimate, sensual zone. Most people like having their feet massaged. To give a proper foot massage, you will need:

1. At least 45 minutes
2. A basin of warm soapy water
3. Two or three soft towels
4. Massage oil.

Begin the massage by playing soft quiet music. Then gently wash one foot with the soapy water. Take your time washing the foot, about five minutes. During washing remember to do the whole foot: the top, bottom and between the toes. Dry the washed foot with one of the towels. Then go to the other foot.

After you have washed and dried both of your partner's feet, put a small amount of massage oil on your hands and begin to massage the left foot. First rub the foot all over, top and bottom, making sure that the whole foot is covered lightly with oil. Then begin at the heel, and massage the bottom of the foot. Use your thumbs and fingers to knead the foot. Slowly work up the bottom of the foot, adding more massage oil if necessary. Remember, this is a gentle massage. Rub gently.

Massage the ball of the foot. Then massage each toe, and between each toe. When you have completed the toes, rub the top of the foot, then gently rub the whole foot. Wipe off any excess oil from your partner's foot. Then go to the right foot and repeat the massage. Take approximately 15 minutes to do each foot.

When you have completed the massage, clean up the area, so that your partner can continue to relax without considering the mess. Allow your partner to lie back and enjoy the experience of being relaxed and nurtured. If you and your partner have decided to swap massages, consider doing them on different days, so the partner being massaged does not have to pay back the massage immediately. Give the massage as a gift of love and caring.

9

Being Clear

One of the major challenges in a relationship is to develop clear and direct communication between partners. For co-dependents this poses a particular problem since they did not learn healthy communication as children. Dysfunctional families communicate only indirectly: with innuendo, partial truths, hints, threats and the withholding of affection. Consequently, the children grow up with the mistaken belief that indirect communication is effective.

Katie, a member of a co-dependency group, explained how she learned to communicate: "My mother would get me to tell my sister, Angela, when Mom was angry at her. She would never tell Angela herself. But, through me, Mom made sure she got the message. Sometimes," Katie continued, "Mom and Angela would be in the same room and my mother would look at me and say, 'Tell your sister I'm angry at her.' Until I was an adult, I never knew there was anything wrong with this. I thought that was the way everybody communicated."

Learning new and healthier kinds of communication is critical for co-dependents. No matter how loving our intentions, an inability to communicate clearly with our partner will become an obstacle in the relationship. Healthy communication transmits information accurately from one partner to the other. For a relationship to be truly intimate, each partner must be able to share truthfully their needs, desires, fears, hopes and joys.

The art of clear communication involves two very important skills: listening and speaking. Most of us believe we already have these skills, but putting them into practice in a recovering relationship requires taking another look at how well we speak and listen, and how we can improve on what we already know.

Listening

To listen well is one of the greatest gifts we can give to our partner. Not all of the ways we listen are loving or helpful. There are three basic types of listening:

1. **Pretend listening**
2. **Passive listening**
3. **Interactive listening**

Pretend Listening

Pretend listening occurs when the listener is not really listening closely. In this case the listener hears only key words and phrases. Using these key words and phrases, they guess at the general message, often misinterpreting it. During pretend listening, the listener plans a reply while their partner is speaking, rather than hear what is being said. When someone is pretend listening, they may interrupt the speaker by injecting comments of their own, sometimes even completing the speaker's sentences for them. Pretend listening is practiced by many people who consider themselves good listeners. It is, however, a very limited way of listening and is disrespectful of the person who is speaking.

One client described her ex-husband as a pretend listener: "He would complete my sentences for me, and sometimes he would be right about what I was going to say. That was so frustrating! I needed to be heard, to say my piece, even if he did sometimes know what I was going to say. I was continually frustrated and angry when I tried to talk to him."

Passive Listening

During passive listening, the listener does not respond but stays passive. They even limit the responses they give through their body language. The passive listener is trying to listen to their partner without becoming emotionally involved in the process. This is an almost impossible task. Partners cannot really become emotionally detached. It is just not the nature of the intimate relationship. The person engaged in passive listening may feel afraid to reveal their own feelings and may use a mask of passivity to cover their fear.

The passive listener may consider themselves very accepting and tolerant of their partner's feelings and expressions. But it is frustrating to talk to a passive listener. One client described his conversations with his passively listening spouse: "Talking to her was like talking into a vacuum. I could never get a response. I never knew whether what I said had any impact on her."

Interactive Listening

Interactive listening involves two-way communication between a speaker and a listener. The listener lets the speaker know they are being heard, even though the listener's response may be as simple as a nod of the head. Their body language and facial expression shows their attentiveness and alertness. Occasionally an interactive listener will ask for restatement or clarification of what has been said. The attitude of the interactive listener is: "I am fully present with you. What you are saying matters to me, and I want to be sure that I understand you correctly."

It is not easy to be an interactive listener. It takes a lot of practice and conscious effort.

John, a recovering co-dependent, related this story about his communication with his wife: "When Helen would talk to me, I would nod my head and smile but I wasn't really paying attention to her. After 10 years of marriage, I thought I had heard everything she had to say. I didn't complete her sentences for her out loud, but I did it silently to myself! I did not realize I was being disrespectful of her. During therapy I started trying to *really hear* what she was saying, and I was very surprised to find out what was really going on with her. Now I really try to let her know that I am listening to her, and when I drift off into my old habit of not paying attention, I tell her what has happened and ask her to repeat what I missed."

Speaking Effectively

Speaking effectively is another communication skill that co-dependents must learn in a recovering relationship. Co-dependents often become frustrated when they are unable to ask their partners for what they want and need. When co-dependents rely on the hints and innuendo they learned in their dysfunctional families, it is almost sure that they will not get exactly what it is they want because their partner has to guess at it. Many co-dependents expect their partner to do mind-reading. When their partner guesses wrongly about what they hinted at, they become angry. The unhealthy belief behind their anger is that, "If you really loved me, you would already know what I want." This expectation is unrealistic. Effective speaking consists of:

> Being Direct
> Being Specific
> Being Brief
> Sending Consistent Messages
> Using "I" Statements

Being Direct

First of all, being direct about needing to take up an issue with our partner involves directly addressing them. A partner who wants to discuss an important matter with their spouse needs to begin by saying, "I want to talk to you." Then the couple can decide whether to talk right away, or to set a more appropriate time when they won't be interrupted. Healthy communication is not done through a third person, such as a friend or child. This habit of indirect communication, so common in dysfunctional families, causes confusion and misunderstanding. Direct, person-to-person communication means taking responsibility for what we have to say to our partner and being personally available to hear their response.

Being Specific

Being specific means stating what we are feeling, thinking or needing as exactly and precisely as we can. The speaker does not hint, and avoids vagueness. When someone is being specific, their partner does not have to guess at what is being communicated. Being specific means making clear statements, avoiding ambiguity.

Here are some examples of confusing, nonspecific statements: "You make me mad," "You are so moody!" "You always make us late." These non-specific statements do not convey constructive information to a partner. Instead their primary message is blame.

Three examples of specific statements are: "I am feeling sad," "I will do the grocery shopping this week," "I would like a hug." Specific statements are simple and direct, and clearly tell our partner exactly what we are feeling, what we need from them or what our plans are. Giving our partner clear messages can prevent hurt feelings and needless disagreements.

Being Brief

Brevity in communication between co-dependents is an asset. When a statement is brief and to-the-point, communication is smoother and the subject of discussion is more memorable. Many co-dependents have difficulty talking about emotionally charged subjects. We may tend to ramble, to bring up other (unrelated) grievances and generally wander from the main topic. For the co-dependent who greatly fears that their partner may respond angrily, such discussions can be very stressful. The co-dependent may forget what they meant to say. Their mind may go blank. The more concisely we state things, the less likelihood there is that we will forget or ramble.

I often suggest writing down feelings and thoughts about the issue before the discussion takes place. (If the talk is planned, both partners may do this.) This helps to keep us focused on the topic.

An example of a brief, direct statement is: "We had an agreement to plan a budget together on Thursday evening. You broke that agreement and I am angry." When making a concise statement like this, it is important to remember that our partner has the right to respond in their own way. If we just make the statement and walk away, we are "dropping a bomb." Communicating responsibly involves being present for our partner's response to what we have said, even if we are resistant to hearing it.

Sending Consistent Messages

During direct face-to-face communication, we transmit information not only by the words we use, but by our tone of voice, facial expression and body posture. As a matter of fact, we say much more with our nonverbal cues than we do with our words. Therefore, it is important not just to say what we mean, but to let our tone of voice, facial expression and body posture reflect the same message we are verbalizing. Our listener will be more likely to believe us if they see the emotional power behind our words. When someone says, "I'm really angry at you," with a smile on their face and a mellow tone of voice, the listener is likely to discount or ignore the statement of anger. If the same person said tersely, "I am so angry at you right now that I feel like I'm going to explode!" there would be little room for the listener to misunderstand the message. I often ask clients to speak in front of a mirror or with another person to practice making their body signals consistent with their words.

Using "I" Statements

Basic to clear communication with our partner is the use of "I" statements. "I" statements indicate that the speaker is taking responsibility for the feelings and thoughts they express, and not just dumping them on their partner. The statement, "I am feeling hurt," is a statement of how one feels. The speaker can continue by explaining how their feelings have been hurt, which is also important to express.

For example: "I am feeling hurt. We had an agreement to spend Sunday together and on Saturday you broke our date to go fishing with James. I really wish you hadn't done that." When a person says, "*You* hurt my feelings," they are not taking responsibility for having their feelings. Such statements cause resentments.

Beware of using false "I" statements. These are statements that may seem like clear "I" statements, but are not: "*I* feel that *you* are angry" is not an expression of what the speaker feels. Rather, it is an expression of what the speaker thinks their *partner* is feeling. Co-dependents often have difficulty using "I" statements because they may view them as selfish or self-centered. In fact, "I" statements honor the speaker's dignity to own their own feelings.

Summary

Being direct, specific and brief, sending consistent messages, and using "I" statements are fundamentals of clear communication. Because honesty and directness are threatening to the dysfunctional family's denial system, co-dependents were unable to learn these communication skills in childhood. For a recovering couple, practicing these skills may well be their most important undertaking. It is important to practice using healthy communication skills in our everyday interactions with each other. If a couple only practices interactive listening and directness when a conflict is taking place, resolving the conflict will be more difficult.

Below are two examples of conversations between couples. In the first example, a couple uses indirect and nonspecific speech. In the second example, the couple uses healthy communication skills.

Joe and Kathy have agreed to go out to dinner:

Joe: What would you like to eat tonight — Chinese food?

Kathy: I don't know. What would you like to eat?

Joe: I don't care. Wherever you want to eat is okay with me.

Kathy: Would you like to eat pizza?

Joe: I don't know. Would you?

The above conversation could go on for a long time without the couple ever deciding where to eat. Kathy and Joe would sooner or later become frustrated. Typically, they would either decide angrily not to go anywhere, or one person would take control and they might end up eating at a restaurant that neither one enjoyed. In this situation, Joe preferred to eat Chinese food and Kathy preferred pizza, but neither communicated their preference clearly and directly. By starting out indirectly, Joe tried to place the responsibility for the evening on Kathy. By suggesting Chinese food in such a way, Joe also tried to manipulate Kathy into saying she wanted the same thing he wanted without his having to state his preference. But Kathy wanted pizza and was using the same tactics on Joe. This example may seem humorous, but it illustrates how even simple decisions can become frustrating for a couple when they habitually communicate indirectly.

The following conversation between Joe and Kathy is clearer and more direct:

Joe: I'd like to eat Chinese food tonight.
Kathy: I'd rather have pizza than Chinese food but my preference isn't that strong.
Joe: I've been looking forward to eating Chinese food all day, and really would like to have it for dinner tonight.
Kathy: Okay, we can have pizza the next time we eat out. Let's go.

In the second example, Joe clearly stated his preference and so did Kathy. Kathy also began a compromise by adding that her preference was not a strong one. Joe negotiated by directly explaining how much he had been looking forward to a Chinese dinner. Their compromise was to postpone having pizza until the next time they ate out. Using clear communication in everyday situations is important. It keeps life simpler and gives the couple practice, so that when more emotionally charged issues arise, they can deal with them in a healthy way.

An Exercise
Talking About Sex

Most co-dependents have difficulty discussing sex clearly and directly. They have difficulty both asking for what they want sexually and listening to the sexual needs and desires of their partner. The following exercise is designed to help couples become clearer and more open with each other about their sexual thoughts, desires and feelings.

An Exercise In Talking About Sex

Below is a series of open-ended statements that focus on sexual perceptions and feelings. Self-disclosure of sexual information is a necessary part of intimacy in your sexual relationship. Becoming more comfortable talking about sexuality in the relationship enriches all dimensions of the relationship, not just the sexual aspect.

Here are some guidelines for doing this exercise:

Take turns being first to complete the statements.
Respond to each statement before continuing to the next statement.
Either partner may decline to answer any statement.
Either partner may end the exercise at any time.

1. I feel my body is . . .
2. The part of my body I like the most is . . .
3. My mother told me sex was . . .
4. My first sexual memory is . . .
5. I think masturbation is . . .
6. When I talk about sex, I . . .
7. My father told me sex was . . .
8. Right now I feel . . .
9. For me sex and emotional involvement is . . .
10. The most sensuous spot on my body is . . .
11. I like it when you touch my . . .
12. I feel sexually turned on when you . . .
13. My genitals are . . .
14. If I don't have an orgasm during sex, I feel . . .

15. If you don't have an orgasm during sex, I . . .
16. The first time I had intercourse, I felt . . .
17. After we make love, I want to . . .
18. When I touch your genitals, I . . .
19. Something I would like to do sexually that we haven't done is . . .
20. I get afraid when . . .
21. I feel sexually inadequate when . . .
22. I don't like it when you . . .
23. I feel most attractive when . . .
24. I feel close to you when . . .
25. When you kiss me, I . . .
26. Something I really like to do sexually is . . .
27. I feel most vulnerable during sex when . . .
28. My sex life with you is . . .
29. My favorite sexual fantasy is . . .
30. Something I haven't asked for sexually is . . .
31. Something new I have learned about you is . . .
32. What I have learned about myself from this experience is . . .
33. Right now my feelings toward you are . . .
34. At this moment I want to . . .
35. Sharing this experience with you has been . . .

Feel free to expand the above exercise by creating your own open-ended statements. People in recovery are constantly involved in change. Doing this experience several times a year can be helpful in staying clear and current with your partner.

10

Dimensions Of Intimacy

Intimacy means different things to different people. It may mean the closeness a parent feels to a child. Someone else may feel their deepest intimate connection with a friend. In the committed sexual relationship, intimacy is having a deep heart-to-heart connection with our partner.

Intimacy does not happen by accident nor does it occur overnight. True intimacy in a relationship is developed over a period of time, as the result of the couple's consistent joint effort. A deeper feeling of intimacy, that wonderful feeling of safety in being ourselves with another person, is one of the greatest benefits of transforming a co-dependent relationship to a recovering relationship.

For any two people to develop intimacy requires work, knowledge and commitment. When both partners come from dysfunctional families, they have the added challenge of overcoming self-defeating behavior patterns and attitudes learned in childhood.

Here it is important to make a distinction between romantic love and intimacy. Romantic love (often the force that first brings a couple together) is intensely exciting and sexually passionate. While we are falling in love, we feel as though we will have this intense excitement with our lover forever. Of course, the fire of romantic love inevitably begins to cool, usually then we are no longer able to ignore our partner's human faults and limitations. It is at this juncture, when romantic love begins to lessen in intensity, that some relationships fall apart. Others may remain intact but become dysfunctional. The excitement of romantic love by itself does not create a healthy intimacy between lovers. However, couples who are interested in building a stronger, more committed relationship can use the experience of romantic love as a foundation for intimacy.

Conscious action by both partners is necessary to develop intimacy. To make this conscious decision requires that we know what it is to be intimate. There are four dimensions of intimacy in committed sexual relationships:

Physical
Emotional
Mental
Spiritual

The recovering couple who want intimacy must bring their efforts to every dimension of life. When we have intimacy with another, we share ourselves on all levels of existence.

We would not think of saying to our spouse or lover, "Now I'm going to express to you my deepest emotions about my spiritual beliefs, but I'm not going to tell you what my spiritual beliefs are." Sharing our feelings without sharing the context of the feelings would be difficult to do and it would certainly confuse our partner. In a healthy relationship these dimensions are not distinct from each other but are integrated into the fabric of the relationship. This integration depends upon the couple's willingness to actively seek intimacy in all four dimensions of their life together. Although the physical, emotional, mental and spiritual dimensions naturally blend and overlap, it is simpler for our purposes to address them separately.

The Physical Dimension

Touching

Human beings need to be touched, held and hugged. Respectful holding and hugging are tender and compassionate acts that create a trusting bond and fulfill a basic human need. This need for touch may be repressed or unacknowledged but it exists in everyone. Being in a healthy relationship is a physical experience. There is a healing power in human touch. The intimate couple can use touch to support and nurture each other.

Partners need to be aware that touching and hugging should not always lead to a sexual experience. In fact, *most* touching in a healthy relationship will not become sexual. Many people from dysfunctional families learned that physical intimacy is always sexual. While sex is a form of physical intimacy, it is only one of *many* forms.

Recovering couples will want to experiment with non-sexual touching, to expand limited beliefs about physical intimacy with each other. Such practice is worth the effort. It frees both partners to physically express their love and tenderness for each other at times when they may not want to have sex.

Boundaries

When two people share the same physical space, issues of privacy and boundaries arise. Most people in Western culture have a need for their own space. It may be a physical space in the apartment or house, a private journal, time away from the relationship to be with friends or time spent in solitude. Whatever form our boundaries take, space and privacy are legitimate needs that deserve our respect.

Each partner needs to be able to establish and maintain physical boundaries. Being in a sexual relationship does not mean that either partner has unlimited access to the other's body. When a partner sets limits on the amount or kind of touching they want or on their sexual availability, they are setting a personal boundary. Setting a boundary is not the same as creating a barrier to intimacy. Our boundaries are important statements about who we are. They signal our preferences and desires. Boundaries have to do with the person who sets the limit and are not a reflection on the character or personality of their partner. Unfortunately co-dependents often interpret their partner's boundaries as a personal rejection.

An important thing to know about boundaries is that they can change. Depending on how safe and secure we feel, we may set stringent boundaries (when we find ourselves in a new situation) or very lax boundaries (when we are feeling safe and comfortable). Not only does a person have the right to create a boundary, but they have the right to change the boundaries they create — a good reason for couples to develop the art of staying current in their communication with each other.

People from dysfunctional families often have difficulty knowing how to set healthy boundaries, and expressing those limits to their partner. The recovering couple will need to experiment both in creating, and in changing their personal boundaries with each other.

Sex

While the joyful and satisfying act of physically making love should not be over-emphasized, we must be aware that sex is a powerful force in a relationship. The shared sexuality of a couple is a creative act that builds intimacy and can bring children into the world. At its healthiest sex is experienced by both people as a bonding of their creativity and life force in a way that increases their trust and caring for each other. It is natural and healthy to enjoy sex and have fun making love.

Because they have received mixed messages about appropriate sexual behavior in the past, both partners in a co-dependent relationship need to find for themselves what is appropriate. Part of maturing as a couple is arriving at sexual boundaries in the context of the relationship. What is sexually exciting and desirable to one couple might be uninteresting or unthinkable to another couple. Exploring each other's sexual desires and wishes is one of the adventures of the recovering relationship. Openly talking with each other about sexual desires demystifies sex and contributes to a couple's ability to feel joyful and free in their lovemaking.

Barbara, a co-dependent and an incest survivor, could not tolerate being hugged or touched except during sexual intercourse. Only while she was having sex could she allow her spouse to show physical tenderness. When her husband tried to hug her at other times, she would feel agitated and tense. Barbara was in therapy and knew that as a child she was hugged before having sexual intercourse with her stepfather. She wanted to change her belief that every hug would lead to sex. She and her partner began to experiment with gently touching and hugging each other without leading into sex. After a period of time Barbara began to feel more in control of her body and to feel that she had a *choice* about whether or not to have sex. Now she can hug and touch without feeling she has to pay a price. Healing together often takes time and practice, but the intimacy it builds is well worth the effort.

The Emotional Dimension

Surviving Conflict

When two people join in a relationship, their needs, desires, hopes and dreams sometimes come into conflict. Expecting a relationship to be completely free of conflict is not realistic. Although conflict is a healthy element of every intimate relationship, most co-dependents feel fearful about disagreements with their partner. In the dysfunctional family of origin, conflict was either a form of combat with a winner and a loser or conflict was ignored completely.

Conflicts can involve a variety of subjects: sex, money, jobs, decisions about whether to have children, how to raise the children we do have, whether to move, where to go on vacations. Most of the areas of our lives can be areas of potential conflict. We may disagree about major or minor decisions we must make as a couple or we may simply have different and conflicting feelings about what is happening between us.

Unresolved conflict can seriously damage a relationship. If we have not learned to deal with our conflicts constructively, they stick around causing constant irritation and decreasing our trust of each other. On the other hand our patience and persistence in learning how to solve problems together is one of the greatest contributors to sharing real intimacy with our life partner. Although most conflict situations are resolvable, in some cases a couple must "agree to disagree." We cannot expect that *all* conflicts will be resolved to the satisfaction of both partners. Healthy communication skills are necessary when we begin to address conflicts as a couple. (Try re-reading the chapter "Being Clear" for a review on communication skills.)

The feelings of fear that most co-dependents have surrounding conflict leads them to believe that conflict is bad for the relationship. The opposite is true. Working through conflict in a relationship indicates that both partners are willing to try to work things out, rather than abandon the relationship at the first sign of trouble. By surviving and resolving conflict together, a couple grow to trust each other and to trust that their relationship is strong enough to endure through challenging times.

Becoming Vulnerable

The last thing that most co-dependent people want to do is to be vulnerable. We have so many hurts left over from childhood, we have learned to protect ourselves from abuse by becoming emotionally numb or shut down. So much effort has gone into our techniques and strategies for keeping ourselves *in*vulnerable! As partners in recovery, we must begin to dismantle the wall of detachment we have built around us. While honoring the strong defenses that helped us survive, we must take down the wall gradually and with gentleness.

Although we may want very much to be vulnerable, most co-dependents do not know how. Our defenses operate at an unconscious level, therefore, we will want to begin to learn how to be vulnerable by observing our reactions to our partner very closely. Our willingness to take emotional risks will increase in time as we learn to understand our defensive reactions and as we continue to practice as a team. When our partners are vulnerable, they are telling us they trust us enough to risk being hurt. This trust is an honor — it is earned by our compassion and by our willingness to reserve judgment.

When we are vulnerable with each other, we allow our partner a view of our innermost self. When we lower the barriers we use to hide our true selves from each other, we can make real emotional contact. Authentic intimacy cannot develop without real emotional contact between partners. As our growth together progresses, mistakes will be made and feelings hurt. During this risky process of trusting, couples must be aware that each time they show gentleness and tolerance to each other it is like putting money in the bank. Our patience with ourselves, with each other and with the recovery process will speed our growth and increase our sense of having a healthy bond.

Sharing Feelings

Sharing feelings is fundamental to making emotional contact and developing intimacy. When we hide our feelings from our partner, we hide our essential selves. If our strong feelings are not expressed, we establish a pattern of secrecy and deceit in the relationship. Once this dysfunctional pattern is established, we find we have more and more difficulty sharing with our partner. When this happens, our secrets prevent us from experiencing the kind of intimacy we deserve. It is best to break this cycle of secrecy before a great degree of resentment and bitterness builds. The longer we keep our feelings secret from our partner (especially when these feelings directly concern him or her), the more betrayed our partner is bound to feel once we finally come across with the truth.

When openness exists between committed partners, there is a feeling of lightness and ease about their relationship. When the recovering couple feel free to express *all* feelings in an atmosphere of acceptance and tolerance, *a deep emotional healing takes place in both people*. Because each person's response to sharing is to try to support and nurture (rather than judge or defend) their bond of intimacy grows better and stronger.

John, who grew up in a dysfunctional family, was continually told by the women in his life that he was emotionally unavailable. He came to therapy able to admit this was a problem for him, but unsure about what to do to change it. In his family upbringing, John had suffered extreme verbal abuse. He had been repeatedly ridiculed as a child. Not surprisingly, John closely guarded his emotions, doing all he could to keep others from knowing his feelings. John began to practice expressing what he was feeling in the safe environment of the therapy group. Then he would go home and experiment by disclosing some of his feelings to his wife, Paula. Gradually John overcame his fear about letting Paula know what he was feeling. Seeing John's courageous risk-taking inspired Paula to share in return. Their relationship together became much richer, more intimate and a lot more fun. Although John acknowledges that he still has a lot to learn about expressing his feelings, the exciting improvement in his marriage has sealed his commitment to continue sharing his feelings, even though it is sometimes difficult.

The Mental Dimension

Shared Value Systems

For partners to have similar values means that they share the same general world view and life philosophy. Having similar values is different from having exactly the same values. How hard that would be and how boring!

The recovering couple arrives at opportunities to learn and grow together precisely when they have different ideas about the same things. It is, however, important for the couple to have a basic understanding and agreement about important aspects of their life together. If one partner values scrupulous honesty, and the other partner enjoys annually deceiving the I.R.S., for example, conflict around this issue is bound to recur. When one partner views sexual fidelity as the most important aspect of the relationship, and the other believes that people who love each other should be able to have multiple sexual partners, then the conflict in their value systems will cause serious problems.

When we hold the same basic set of values in common with our partner, each of us can feel confident that our partner will behave in ways that generally agree with what we believe is right. Sadly, many couples rarely talk to each other about what is really of value to them in their lives. Co-dependents often assume they share the same value system with their partners, then are shocked when their partner does something that they consider unthinkable. Discussion and disclosure about personal values prevents each partner from having to do guesswork in this important area. Because recovering partners will change over time, it is important to update each other on new ideas and outlooks that may affect our individual value systems.

A Common Life Plan

Though most of us who are in recovery strive to live "one day at a time," there is nothing wrong with thinking and planning. Financial goals, timing a move for a change in employment and starting a family are all important life events that advance planning can help to happen more smoothly and with less strain on the relationship. Developing a common life plan for the relationship can assist both partners in achieving their personal goals and wishes and can create a direction for the growth of the relationship itself. When we create a blueprint, we are often prevented from making unwise choices on the spur of the moment. Planning together makes it much more likely that our dreams will come true.

Mapping out our future as a couple and living one day at a time can easily coexist. Doing both simply requires that both partners agree to practice flexibility about their plan. The recovering couple can create a plan together, then begin to take steps to put it into action. The couple must also remain conscious that circumstances may change which would require a new plan or would require changes in the existing plan. Sharing a life plan can reduce the stress of living in a changing world. It is important, however, not to become so fixed on seeing our plan materialize that it becomes more important than the people who designed it. If we stay aware of the potential for our rigid thinking to cause us problems, we will be more likely to be open to changes that may occur.

A long-range plan is subject to review at any time by either partner. As the relationship grows and transforms, our dreams and goals will change. Continually updating our life plans in the light of our changing attitudes and desires maintains our sense of teamwork about the life we are creating for ourselves.

Conscious Living

Conscious living means being alert and aware during the ordinary and miraculous process of day-to-day living. Most of us have experienced what it feels like to be taken for granted by someone else. Staying conscious in our relationship includes small kindnesses and creative attentions, such as compliments, surprise gifts and noticing our partner's positive efforts in recovery. Living consciously with another person requires the same, or greater, expenditure of energy and time we would expect to give any other major undertaking. We must *really see* each other, not just glance across the dinner table or the kids. We must *consciously speak* to each other, not just make the same small talk day after day. And we must *creatively play* together, not just sit next to each other at the movies week after week. It is easy to get caught up in the busy rush of all there is to do and forget to stop and acknowledge each other. When this happens, we are taking our relationship for granted.

As a couple consciously involved with each other, we continually renew our commitment and enthusiasm about sharing our lives together. We can never totally know our partner. For this reason, no matter how long we live together, if we do so consciously, we can continue to delight and surprise each other. Special to the recovering co-dependent relationship is our ability to watch, recognize and be amazed by our own and our partner's subtle growth and development in recovery.

Jane, a recovering co-dependent, was in a five-year relationship in which she was relatively happy. She had never realized she had begun to take her partner for granted until one night she realized that, when she looked at her husband, she really did not *see* him. She just looked around him, and she really didn't listen to him when he spoke to her. She heard his words but did not pay very close attention.

She remarked to her therapy group, "I never realized that we were drifting apart. Things were really comfortable between us. We had both done a lot of growing. We just stopped paying attention to each other. Now I can see that it almost cost us our relationship. We were becoming more and more distant. Now we are so much closer: talking, playing, really enjoying each other. It might sound corny, but it's like we're falling in love all over again."

The Spiritual Dimension

Awareness

An awareness of the existence of a Higher Power or some form of spiritual essence is basic to the continuation of recovery in a committed relationship. When each partner is aware of a force or power that transcends the human experience and encompasses all things, then the couple has a source of strength that is powerful and healing. A spiritual presence in our relationship keeps us from relying exclusively on our human partner for strength and compassion. During trying times, the physical, emotional and mental dimensions of intimacy with our partner may not be enough to comfort us and help us feel safe. At such times the spiritual aspect of our commitment to each other binds us together until our circumstances stabilize again.

Practice

Although each member of the relationship does not have to follow the same spiritual path, it is important that the couple have a spiritual practice that they do together. This spiritual practice could be going to a worship service, meditating, praying or working a 12-step program together. Whatever we choose, the importance of sharing our spiritual practice (or parts of it) as a couple cannot be overemphasized. When a couple consciously does a spiritual practice together, a very strong bond forms between them. This spiritual bond exists soul-to-soul and cannot be broken by external events. True soulmates are bonded at the spiritual level. Our regular and consistent spiritual practice together both creates and strengthens this magical bond.

Service

Essential to a spiritual way of life is to be of service in the world. The couple that is spiritually bonded usually contributes to their community in some way. Each couple chooses their own form of service work together. This work may appear ordinary, such as lovingly raising healthy children, or it may appear unique, such as becoming a missionary couple. Each of us finds in our heart our decision about how to be of service. It is part of the work of the relationship to make room for both individuals to do the kind of service work they feel guided to do. It is important, however, that some aspect of this service is a shared commitment. When we strive to become healthy and happy as a recovering couple, one of the most satisfying fruits of our labor is to share our experience of growth and health with others in recovery.

There is a saying in 12-step programs: "You can't keep what you have found unless you give it away." Just as the recovering individual must share their new-found health, recovering couples must also pass it on.

A great teacher once remarked that if we live in a relationship for many years, our partner changes in so many ways, it is like being married to three or four different people! He also said that if we do not recognize and cherish the changes in our partner, then we are spiritually asleep, and will not be able to enjoy the full experience of our marriage.

The four dimensions of intimacy are to guide the recovering couple in building trust and intimacy together. They are not to be used to judge whether the relationship is passing or failing a test. It is our humanness that sparks the passion and joy in relationships, and our humanity is the greatest gift we can give each other, including all the mistakes and errors of judgment that human beings are prone to make.

If your relationship falls short of your ideal fantasy, you're in good company. Be gentle — allow yourself and your partner room to grow and change. If you attempt to stay conscious of them as a couple, the four dimensions of intimacy can provide a basis for deep compassion between you and your partner.

Staying conscious in a relationship is not *all* work. It should be fun, too! Below is a list of warm fuzzies (*warm fuzzies* help a person feel warm, cozy, and loved). These are gifts for you and your partner to share. Copy each warm fuzzy onto a 3 X 5 card (create your own *warm fuzzies*, too). You may give the coupons to your partner one at a time, or all at once. When your partner needs a "warm fuzzy," they can turn in a coupon. The coupons may also be split up so that each partner starts out with 15 coupons to redeem. However you decide to set it up, the most important part of giving and receiving "warm fuzzies" is having fun and letting your partner know that you care.

Warm Fuzzy Coupons
(gifts for the one you love)

When you turn in this coupon,
I will surprise you some time
this week with a bouquet of flowers.

This coupon is good for
one 30-minute
back rub.

This gift certificate
is redeemable
for breakfast in bed.

This coupon will be honored
for one treat
to an afternoon movie.

A gift coupon of
one 45-minute
foot massage (with oil).

A coupon for
one free car wash
(inside and out).

This coupon is redeemable for
one "I love you" telephone call
a day for one week.

Redeemable for a romantic evening
for two at the
restaurant of your choice.

Good for one picnic:
I get the food,
you pick the place.

A coupon for one walk,
holding hands,
lasting at least 45 minutes.

A gift certificate for a morning
of being your chauffeur, and driving
you wherever you want to go.

When you turn in this certificate,
you will receive one full body massage
lasting at least one hour.

With this coupon you will receive
a birthday card on a day
that is not your birthday.

This coupon entitles you
to a 30-minute massage on the part
of your body of your choice.

Redeemable for one two-minute hug,
three times a day,
for five days.

Redeemable for
one surprise gift
of my choice.

Good for one hour of snuggling
at the time and place
of your choice.

Redeemable for
one prepared bubble bath
and a back wash.

Turn in this coupon and I
will read you any poem or story
you ask me to read.

Redeemable for
watching a sunrise or
a sunset with you.

With this coupon
you will receive four
surprise hugs, with kisses.

With this coupon you will receive
an afternoon of playing together
(you pick the games).

This coupon is good
for one hour of watching the
moon and stars together.

This coupon is redeemable for one evening
by yourself. (I'll watch the kids, cats, dogs or
do whatever is necessary for you to be alone.)

When you turn in this coupon,
I will look into your eyes
and tell you that I love you.

This is an appreciation coupon:
When you redeem this, I will tell you
five reasons why I appreciate you.

Good for one coloring book,
crayons and a
coloring companion (me).

Redeemable for a trip to the park,
a push on the swings and
a partner on the see-saw.

Good for a one-hour guided body massage
(you guide the massage)
complete with music, low lights and oil.

This coupon is good for
one evening of
hanging out and having fun.

Conclusion

The journey of recovery from co-dependence is always (at least in part) a difficult and frightening experience. When you choose to include a life partner on your journey, the task of recovering may begin to appear even more difficult and complex. But this is not the case. By definition, recovery from co-dependence happens within the context of human relationships. Recovery does not occur in isolation. To recover from co-dependence, we need people in our lives. The committed sexual relationship holds abundant opportunities, both for becoming aware of co-dependent issues and for resolving them. Having a solid recovering relationship is a great asset not a liability.

The support and love that you and your partner offer each other will contribute greatly to the healing process. When two people focus together on love and understanding through the process of recovering from the wounds of childhood, they create a place of safety where both partners can truly heal together. Because we must be transformed by our recovery, the path of the recovering couple leads not only to love and intimacy, but also to spiritual fulfillment. Couples who persevere on this journey will be the beneficiaries of an ever-changing experience that is wonderful, joyful and enlightening. Our peaceful future in the world depends on how well we are able to compromise, to negotiate, to consciously love each other. For all of us, these skills must start at home where, by meeting conflict with courage and loving kindness, we break the cycle and begin to heal together.

Bibliography

Bass, Ellen and Davis, Laura. **The Courage to Heal.** New York: Harper & Row, 1988.

Bradshaw, John. **Bradshaw On: Healing The Shame That Binds You.** Deerfield Beach, Florida: Health Communications, 1988.

Campbell, Joseph with Moyers, Bill. **The Power of Myth.** New York: Doubleday, 1988.

Chang, Jolan. **The Tao of the Loving Couple.** New York: E.P. Dutton, 1983.

Douglas, Nik and Slinger, Penny. **Sexual Secrets.** New York: Destiny Books, 1979.

Haldane, Sean. **Couple Dynamics.** Far Hills, New Jersey: New Horizon Press, 1985.

Johnson, Robert A. **We: Understanding the Psychology of Romantic Love.** San Francisco: Harper & Row, 1983.

Mandel, Bob. **Two Hearts Are Better Than One.** Berkeley, California: Celestial Arts, 1986.

Masters, William H.; Johnson, Virginia E. and Kolodny, Robert C. **Masters and Johnson on Sex and Human Loving.** Boston: Little, Brown and Company, 1986.

Pfeiffer, J. William and Jones, John E., eds. **A Handbook of Structured Experiences for Human Relations Training,** Vol. V, "Dyadic

Renewal: A Program for Developing Ongoing Relationships," San Diego, California: University Associates, 1975.

Scarf, Maggie. **Intimate Partners.** New York: Random House, 1987.

Vissell, Barry and Vissell, Joyce. **The Shared Heart.** Aptos, California: Ramira Publishing, 1984.

Woititz, Janet G. **Healing Your Sexual Self.** Deerfield Beach: Health Communications, 1989.

――――――. **Struggle For Intimacy.** Pompano Beach: Health Communications, 1985.

Books from . . .
Health Communications

AFTER THE TEARS: Reclaiming The Personal Losses of Childhood
Jane Middelton-Moz and Lorie Dwinnel
Your lost childhood must be grieved in order for you to recapture your
self-worth and enjoyment of life. This book will show you how.
ISBN 0-932194-36-2   **$7.95**

HEALING YOUR SEXUAL SELF
Janet Woititz
How can you break through the aftermath of sexual abuse and enter into
healthy relationships? Survivors are shown how to recognize the problem
and deal effectively with it.
ISBN 1-55874-018-X   **$7.95**

RECOVERY FROM RESCUING
Jacqueline Castine
Effective psychological and spiritual principles teach you when to take
charge, when to let go, and how to break the cycle of guilt and fear that
keeps you in the responsibility trap. Mind-altering ideas and exercises will
guide you to a more carefree life.
ISBN 1-55874-016-3   **$7.95**

ADDICTIVE RELATIONSHIPS: Reclaiming Your Boundaries
Joy Miller
We have given ourselves away to spouse, lover, children, friends or
parents. By examining where we are, where we want to go and how to get
there, we can reclaim our personal boundaries and the true love of
ourselves.
ISBN 1-55874-003-1   **$7.95**

RECOVERY FROM CO-DEPENDENCY:
It's Never Too Late To Reclaim Your Childhood
Laurie Weiss, Jonathan B. Weiss
Having been brought up with life-repressing decisions, the adult child
recognizes something isn't working. This book shows how to change
decisions and live differently and fully.
ISBN 0-932194-85-0   **$9.95**

SHIPPING/HANDLING: All orders shipped UPS unless weight exceeds 200 lbs., special routing is requested, or
delivery territory is outside continental U.S. Orders outside United States shipped either Air Parcel Post or Surface
Parcel Post. Shipping and handling charges apply to all orders shipped whether UPS, Book Rate, Library Rate, Air
or Surface Parcel Post or Common Carrier and will be charged as follows. Orders less than $25.00 in value add
$2.00 minimum. Orders from $25.00 to $50.00 in value (after discount) add $2.50 minimum. Orders greater than
$50.00 in value (after discount) add 6% of value. Orders greater than $25.00 outside United States add 15% of
value. We are not responsible for loss or damage unless material is shipped UPS. Allow 3-5 weeks after receipt of
order for delivery. Prices are subject to change without prior notice.

Enterprise Center, 3201 S.W. 15th Street,
Deerfield Beach, FL 33442
1-800-851-9100

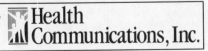 **Health Communications, Inc.**

Other Books By . . .
Health Communications, Inc.

ADULT CHILDREN OF ALCOHOLICS
Janet Woititz
Over a year on *The New York Times* Best-Seller list, this book is the primer on Adult Children of Alcoholics.
ISBN 0-932194-15-X $6.95

STRUGGLE FOR INTIMACY
Janet Woititz
Another best-seller, this book gives insightful advice on learning to love more fully.
ISBN 0-932194-25-7 $6.95

DAILY AFFIRMATIONS: *For Adult Children of Alcoholics*
Rokelle Lerner
These positive affirmations for every day of the year paint a mental picture of your life as you choose it to be.
ISBN 0-932194-27-3 $6.95

CHOICEMAKING: *For Co-dependents, Adult Children and Spirituality Seekers* — Sharon Wegscheider-Cruse
This useful book defines the problems and solves them in a positive way.
ISBN 0-932194-26-5 $9.95

LEARNING TO LOVE YOURSELF: *Finding Your Self-Worth*
Sharon Wegscheider-Cruse
"Self-worth is a choice, not a birthright", says the author as she shows us how we can choose positive self-esteem.
ISBN 0-932194-39-7 $7.95

BRADSHAW ON: THE FAMILY: *A Revolutionary Way of Self-Discovery*
John Bradshaw
The host of the nationally televised series of the same name shows us how families can be healed and individuals can realize full potential.
ISBN 0-932194-54-0 $9.95

HEALING THE CHILD WITHIN:
Discovery and Recovery for Adult Children of Dysfunctional Families
Charles Whitfield
Dr. Whitfield defines, describes and discovers how we can reach our Child Within to heal and nurture our woundedness.
ISBN 0-932194-40-0 $8.95

Enterprise Center, 3201 S.W. 15th Street,
Deerfield Beach, FL 33442
1-800-851-9100

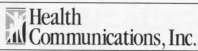
Health Communications, Inc.

Daily Affirmation Books from . . .
Health Communications

GENTLE REMINDERS FOR CO-DEPENDENTS: Daily Affirmations
Mitzi Chandler
With insight and humor, Mitzi Chandler takes the co-dependent and the adult child through the year. Gentle Reminders is for those in recovery who seek to enjoy the miracle each day brings.
ISBN 1-55874-020-1   **$6.95**

TIME FOR JOY: Daily Affirmations
Ruth Fishel
With quotations, thoughts and healing energizing affirmations these daily messages address the fears and imperfections of being human, guiding us through self-acceptance to a tangible peace and the place within where there is *time for joy.*
ISBN 0-932194-82-6   **$6.95**

CRY HOPE: Positive Affirmations For Healthy Living
Jan Veltman
This book gives positive daily affirmations for seekers and those in recovery. Everyday is a new adventure, and change is a challenge.
ISBN 0-932194-74-5   **$6.95**

SAY YES TO LIFE: Daily Affirmations For Recovery
Father Leo Booth
These meditations take you through the year day by day with Father Leo Booth, looking for answers and sometimes discovering that there are none. Father Leo tells us, "For the recovering compulsive person God is too important to miss — may you find Him now."
IBN 0-932194-46-X   **$6.95**

DAILY AFFIRMATIONS: For Adult Children of Alcoholics
Rokelle Lerner
Affirmations are a way to discover personal awareness, growth and spiritual potential, and self-regard. Reading this book gives us an opportunity to nurture ourselves, learn who we are and what we want to become.
ISBN 0-932194-47-3
(Little Red Book)   **$6.95**
(New Cover Edition)   **$6.95**

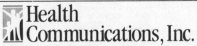

Enterprise Center, 3201 S.W. 15th Street,
Deerfield Beach, FL 33442
1-800-851-9100
Health Communications, Inc.

New Books . . .
from Health Communications

HEALING THE SHAME THAT BINDS YOU
John Bradshaw
Toxic shame is the core problem in our compulsions, co-dependencies and addictions. The author offers healing techniques to help release the shame that binds us.
ISBN 0-932194-86-9 $9.95

THE MIRACLE OF RECOVERY:
Healing For Addicts, Adult Children and Co-dependents
Sharon Wegscheider-Cruse
Beginning with recognizing oneself as a survivor, it is possible to move through risk and change to personal transformation.
ISBN 1-55874-024-4 $9.95

CHILDREN OF TRAUMA: *Rediscovering Your Discarded Self*
Jane Middelton-Moz
This beautiful book shows how to discover the source of past traumas and grieve them to grow into whole and complete adults.
ISBN 1-55874-014-7 $9.95

New Books on Spiritual Recovery . . .

LEARNING TO LIVE IN THE NOW: *6-Week Personal Plan To Recovery*
Ruth Fishel
The author gently introduces you step by step to the valuable healing tools of meditation, positive creative visualization and affirmations.
ISBN 0-932194-62-1 $7.95

CYCLES OF POWER: *A User's Guide To The Seven Seasons of Life*
Pamela Levin
This innovative book unveils the process of life as a cyclic pattern, providing strategies to use the seven seasons to regain power over your life.
ISBN 0-932194-75-3 $9.95

MESSAGES FROM ANNA: *Lessons in Living (Santa Claus, God and Love)*
Zoe Rankin
This is a quest for the meaning of "love." In a small Texas Gulf Coast town a wise 90-year-old woman named Anna shares her life messages.
ISBN 1-55874-013-9 $7.95

THE FLYING BOY: *Healing The Wounded Man*
John Lee
A man's journey to find his "true masculinity" and his way out of co-dependent and addictive relationships, this book is about feelings — losing them, finding them, expressing them.
ISBN 1-55874-006-6 $7.95

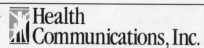

Enterprise Center, 3201 S.W. 15th Street,
Deerfield Beach, FL 33442
1-800-851-9100

Health Communications, Inc.

Helpful 12-Step Books from . . .
Health Communications

HEALING A BROKEN HEART:
12 Steps of Recovery for Adult Children
Kathleen W.

This useful 12-Step book is presently the number one resource for all Adult Children support groups.

ISBN 0-932194-65-6   **$7.95**

12 STEPS TO SELF-PARENTING For Adult Children
Philip Oliver-Diaz and Patricia A. O'Gorman

This gentle 12-Step guide takes the reader from pain to healing and self-parenting, from anger to forgiveness, and from fear and despair to recovery.

ISBN 0-932194-68-0   **$7.95**

THE 12-STEP STORY BOOKLETS
Mary M. McKee

Each beautifully illustrated booklet deals with a step, using a story from nature in parable form. The 12 booklets (one for each step) lead us to a better understanding of ourselves and our recovery.

ISBN 1-55874-002-3   **$8.95**

WITH GENTLENESS, HUMOR AND LOVE:
A 12-Step Guide for Adult Children in Recovery
Kathleen W. and Jewell E.

Focusing on adult child issues such as reparenting the inner child, self-esteem, intimacy and feelings, this well-organized workbook teaches techniques and tools for the 12-step recovery programs.

ISBN 0-932194-77-X   **$7.95**

GIFTS FOR PERSONAL GROWTH & RECOVERY
Wayne Kritsberg

A goldmine of positive techniques for recovery (affirmations, journal writing, visualizations, guided meditations, etc.), this book is indispensable for those seeking personal growth.

ISBN 0-932194-60-5   **$6.95**

Enterprise Center, 3201 S.W. 15th Street,
Deerfield Beach, FL 33442
1-800-851-9100

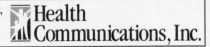

Health Communications, Inc.

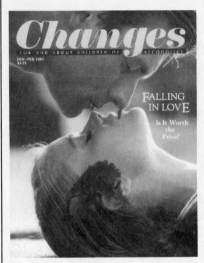